CW00704688

Copyright
Alex Cem

FIRST EDITION

www.alexcem.com

Contents Page

Introduction: Why is *The Six-Pack Mind* Important?

"If you do what you've always done, you'll get what you've always gotten." - Tony Robbins

The Six-Pack Mind is the most in depth exploration of how our psychology affects our physical bodies. *The Six-Pack Mind* will improve your ability to develop the kind of body and health that you want and deserve. Physical transformation is more mental and emotional than we may think. This book consists of some of the most powerful mental and physical tools to help us transform our minds and bodies permanently. Society's current problem is not so much a lack of knowledge, as most of us know how we should eat and exercise. In this book we will predominantly focus on transforming our mental and emotional patterns and thus our behaviours. *The Six-Pack Mind* is about making us the best versions of ourselves. Fortunately, the strategies outlined in this book will make anyone, regardless of current mentality and physical shape, feel and look better. Also, *The Six-Pack Mind* consists of psychological tools to ensure that we deliver, and that our minds are more receptive to our suggestions. *The Six-Pack Mind* will make us feel so much more confident, knowledgeable and in control, so that we avoid unnecessary heartache, frustration and self-deprecation.

Fortunately, in this book, I am going to show you how to take control of your life, how to think, feel and behave, so that you can make the most of your skills and strengths whilst avoiding the pitfalls that most people not only fall into, but live without even knowing it. This book breaks mental, emotions and physical processes down into a granular level, so that you can examine yourself, and transform yourself into the best possible you. The principles in this book are universal, and pertinent to anyone, at any stage in life. You will not only develop yourself tremendously, but you will also inspire those around you; you will have a stronger influence on people because of your newly formed mental, emotional and physical attributes. Genuinely, I look forward to hearing about how *The Six-Pack Mind* has helped you to create the body you have always wanted as well as hearing about the fantastic momentum generated to make other aspects of your life even more wonderful.

Who should read *The Six-Pack Mind?* Anyone who wants to develop their self-esteem, their mind, their emotions and subsequently their body should make use of this book's outstanding content. Why did I decide to write *The Six-Pack Mind?* This book has been created to end the frustration and disappointment people frequently endure in their lives especially as it relates to their health and physical appearance. This book is a meticulous guide that breaks down how we operate internally (so that they can also improve their external world) and why it happens. The purpose of this book is to empower you to appreciate what you have, and to learn about the tools you can utilise to transform mind and body. Passionately, I wanted to communicate all of my knowledge about the psychological aspects of healthy eating, training and overcoming adversity. Painfully, I have seen many people really struggle to control their emotions, especially around eating and exercise, and I have seen them battle unsuccessfully by trying to use willpower alone to surmount their seemingly uncontrollable drive to eat and live in unsupportive ways. Honestly, I was not always adept at controlling my own emotions, focusing on the right things and being consistent. I too have been significantly overweight; I have tried pretty much every diet plan out there, and I have learned that it is not the diet that helps us to remain strong in both mind and body, it is our psychology. I do not have sugar cravings as much as I used to, and if I do, then I have a plethora of strategies to draw upon to keep me on track.

"Pareto's Law can be summarized as follows:
80% of the outputs
result from 20% of the inputs." - Tim Ferriss

I am a massive proponent of Pareto's 80/20 principle as it is applicable to so many different areas in life. In the context of this particular book, I would say that 80% of our success with sustained fat loss is based on our psychology, and only 20% is down to our mechanics (the things that we physically do). We will be looking in great depth into your psychology (80% of this book), and then we will explore the mechanics (20% of this book) as these factors are still highly significant. In the first ten chapters, we will be exploring how to directly affect our self-esteem, beliefs and ability. These fundamental facets will work synergistically to make us happier, which will enable us to attract all the abundance that we want in order to feel complete (and not look for food to fill the incompleteness we feel inside). The final two chapters explore some of the very powerful strategies and habitual practices necessary to ensure that we consistently make better choices. I know that some of us will want to jump straight to the physical tactics we can use, but I urge us to first focus on our psychology (what we think about ourselves, our ability, what stresses us and our relationships with all aspects surrounding healthy eating and training), as this is by far more significant. Have you ever done something in pretty much the same way as someone else, but you both had different results? The key difference here is belief: our psychology.

How can I add value? *The Six-Pack Mind* is almost two decades in the making; it encompasses almost twenty years of studying psychology, communication, leadership, NLP (neuro- linguistic programming) and how to influence ourselves. *The Six-Pack Mind* consists of my own experiences and essential mental programming that I am happy to share with you, so that you can also achieve your dreams (and not just physically). Even though I am a successful, happy person with high self-esteem, it was not always the case. In fact, I used to be an overweight and unfit person, and after years of training and conditioning my mind to perceive food and exercise healthily, I now have a completely natural, strong and attractive body. Proudly, I feel qualified to write about how to transform both mind and body as it relates to health and the body for many reasons: firstly, I am an experienced, certified personal trainer; secondly, I have naturally transformed from an overweight person into someone who consistently has a strong and ripped body without the use of any illicit drugs (and I live in the UK, so you must appreciate that the weather is not always on my side); thirdly, in terms of having a six pack, I have the most challenging body type genetically as I am primarily an endomorph (someone who tends to gain weight and muscle quite easily), and so I have had to dig deeper than most (those with leaner body types, and those who use superior physically enhancing supplements) in order to achieve the body and health I really want. Furthermore, whilst much of the information in the book is scientifically proven, many of the things outlined are also based on opinion. Feel free to agree with some notions, and disagree with others. As long as you take many insightful ideas and information from this book, then I am happy to have served you.

Before we explore the different strategies and tools that will enable us to transform mind, body and health, we need to understand *why* we want to do this. As Tony Robbins says, "Having a powerful enough why will provide you with the necessary how." We must consider the feelings we will get from being able to develop the mind and body we have always wanted, and to keep them this way! Why do you want a better-looking body? Why do you want to live more healthily? What will get you out of bed with energy, and what will keep you on the right track when things are not going smoothly? Is it because you want to spend the rest of your life with a fabulous partner? Is it because you want to finally conquer something that has always been bothering you? Is it so that you can live for longer, and not be restricted in movement in your later life? Is it so that you can set a great example for your children, siblings, peers and so on? Decide now.

We live in a world that is becoming ever more complicated, where the stakes are higher and patience is lower. Our busy lifestyles result in many issues that ruin our ability to feel truly happy, and thus we make more irrational decisions, oftentimes detrimentally affecting our bodies and health. Technological advancements, increasing demands in the workplace, and impatient people make it harder than ever to work on yourself. We must know how we operate, what we can do and why we should do them. Regardless of what we think we are after, all we really want is to experience a need. Think about it, if you want a great body, then you really want to feel accepted whether it is by people on the beach or by your partner or by yourself. If you want to hopefully live a long life without much physical pain, then you are looking for certainty; you want to control your destiny. If you want to feel physically adept, flexible and strong in a physical endeavour, then you want to feel significant. Obviously these feelings correlate to some extent. We all need these feelings continuously (significance, love, certainty and variety as Tony Robbins shares), but one or two of them take precedence. Also, people experience different feelings from different situations. For example, some people get variety from the food they eat, and so the feelings they want to get from their intimate relationship is one of certainty and stability. Some people may get their feelings of significance from their careers, and so the feelings they want to get from food is one of love and connection (yes, we can be connected with food in many ways: instant gratification; when eating out with other people, and we want to build rapport etc.). Take a moment to consider what you currently want to get from food, and readjust your perceptions and lifestyle as necessary.

The key to making the most of the content within this book is to apply it within your life as soon as possible. We need an open mindset when reading *The Six-Pack Mind* because we may come across some unfamiliar notions, or we may believe that some of these concepts are too meticulous and unnecessary. Just read it, and give it a go! Carol Dweck teaches that there are two types of people: those with a fixed mindset and those with a growth mindset (both can be successful, but those with growth mindsets tend to really maximise their potential). Those with a fixed mindset are unable to change and consider their abilities, and others', anew because deep down they believe they cannot improve their minds and bodies significantly. Those with a growth mindset know that they can always do better if they have the desire, work ethic and support necessary. Please readjust your state now to ensure you have the right mentality to absorb this information, and to take immediate action to implement them into your lifestyle.

You will need to read this book several times if you are to really embed the core principles to help you take control of your inner and outer world. Learn how to direct your thoughts. Understand how your emotions work. You will notice your self-esteem improve drastically as a result of your increasing self-acceptance and self-appreciation. You will notice how things do not bother you like they used to bother you. You will be able to change your mood more quickly, and shift your focus toward more empowering notions by improving your emotional intelligence. I am truly grateful to be part of this journey with you. I promise to give you the knowledge needed to direct your thoughts, emotions and actions to areas that will fulfil you. All I need is your commitment and determination to adhere to the notions and principles outlined in this book. Your energy is essential, and you need to take action as of now. Time does not wait for anyone. Let us begin now.

"I have been impressed with the urgency of doing. Knowing is not enough; we must apply. Being willing is not enough; we must do."
- Leonardo da Vinci

Chapter 1: Psychology – Blueprints and Thresholds

"It is not until you change your identity to match your life blueprint that you will understand why everything in the past never worked." – Shannon L. Alder

We have blueprints for many different areas in our lives. We all have certain standards as it relates to our careers, how our relationships must be, how much wealth we should have and so on. Also, we have blueprints as it relates to our physical bodies. This means that we are content with our body once it looks a certain way. Some extreme athletes and bodybuilders have unrealistic expectations of how good their bodies must be, which is why they are never fully satisfied with their bodies because they are chasing the impossible: perfection. This mentality can actually work for them because it keeps them hungry. However, for most people, this mentality will not work because of the pressure of constantly getting better, even if our bodies were fantastic, is too great and intense. People have different blueprints for their physical appearances. For example, a body builder's blueprint may be to only have 5% body fat whereas a previously overweight person's blueprint may be to have 25% body fat. These different people have different priorities and expectations as to how they should look most often.

11

Blueprints can be changed depending on our feelings of competence in these areas.

The problem occurs when we have really awful blueprints! Think of your blueprint as being a robust elastic band. When you pull the elastic band apart, there will be a time when there is so much resistance that the elastic band will snap back to its standard size. This is how our blueprints work. We may go astray every now and then, but our internal resistance will bring us back to our blueprints. It does not matter whether we are bodybuilders or belly builders, we all react the same way whenever we go above or below our blueprints. If we currently have a body that actually looks better than what we really envision for ourselves permanently, then we will, consciously or subconsciously, become more laid back and less disciplined in order to find our way back to the norm. We may start to think things like, "Well I am in good shape now, so I guess I can have that cake now even though it is not my cheat day." "Do I really have to get up at 5 this morning? I mean, I look and feel pretty great. I think I am going to have a lie in today." Conversely, if we fall below our physical blueprint, then we will become very motivated to get back on track: we will become more incensed, focused and driven in order to get back to our acceptable physical condition.

What is your current physical blueprint? How do you expect to look? What do you expect to weigh? How do you expect to move? Let us take this to the next level. What would your body look like if you doubled the quality of your current physical expectations? This now needs to become your new physical blueprint. You now need to associate with this new blueprint: take a moment to imagine yourself looking into the mirror, appreciating your physique as you turn around to see different angles of this new, stronger, healthy-looking you. Zoom in on the beautiful aspects of this new body. Look at the joy in your face. This is the new standard. What can you do to achieve this result, and what can you do to sustain this new you? What type of meals will you consistently need to eat? How often do you need to exercise to maintain this body and health? What will you need to buy? How will this alter the contents within your wardrobe? In order to be able to travel to our new destination, we must know where we currently are.

Your Personal Balance Sheet

"Will you have been an asset or a liability on the world's balance sheet?" – Ryan Lilly

We must spend more time working on what we cannot see, and consequentially we will have incredible physical lives. The problem is most people chase what they can see (house, car, clothes, trophy partner etc.), and so these people often lack the emotional and mental fortitude needed to truly be content and happy. We must believe that we deserve more. We get what we consistently and congruently ask for in life. Now is a fantastic opportunity to reflect. Why do you deserve this new and incredible body? Why is it important to you? How will you feel when you achieve this physique? How will your mentality change when you are able to maintain this sensational shape? What do you currently do very well? Where do you currently let yourself down? A traditional balance sheet is a statement of the assets, liabilities, and capital of a business. We should also have our own personal balance sheet, so that we can accurately evaluate what our current life looks like.

Firstly, let us look at our mental 'income.' What quality material do you have enter your mind every single day, week or month? What types of people do you regularly listen to? Who are your models and mentors when it comes to your body and mind? Is it a family member, a person trainer, someone inspirational with whom you listen to on YouTube etc.? If you do not have role models in these areas (people who are living your physical dreams), then you do not have quality, empowering knowledge entering your mind on a regular basis. How can you possibly expect to develop in an area where you do not regularly hear inspirational, brilliant notions and information around health and fat loss? It is the same as wanting to be wealthy, yet only listening to poorer people all the time. It just does not make sense.

Secondly, what are your mental and emotional assets? Your assets are what make you rich (mentally and emotionally). What sources make you think and feel better? These are our musts. You must make time for these things. For example, what beliefs do you hold that make you a great person? What emotional states do you access in order to get the best out of yourself? Your beliefs will determine how you perceive physical goals, the mind and body connection, and what you are capable of achieving. Your 'income' (what you have enter your mind consistently) will infiltrate your assets and change your beliefs. We become what we consistently listen to and tell ourselves. Our assets (beliefs) must therefore support us. Here are some examples of quality assets: "I believe that I am in control of my actions." "I believe that my ideal body shape will make me a happier and more successful person in all avenues." "I believe that the body reflects the mind." "I am a constantly improving and determined person especially when it comes to my health and body." "I am responsible for what my body looks and feels like." Your assets will serve to empower you, and keep you on the right track. Consider these and adapt where necessary.

Thirdly, we must ruminate over our expenses. These are the people we listen to every week or month who, in one way or another, detract from our body shape and health goals. These are the people we listen to or people who affect our actions regularly. They are usually family members, friends, peers or society's ideologies. These people might directly say harmful things to us to demoralise us, or they may be people with whom we love who indirectly negatively affect our health and body-shape goals. Here are some examples of what expenses sound like: "Let's all go out for burgers and beer tonight." "You put too much pressure on yourself to lose weight. Just chill out a little." "Your genetics aren't the best, so you'll never get the kind of body you want." "Having a six-pack is not important. Don't you have important things to focus on?" We must ensure that our income outweighs our expenses.

Lastly, we have liabilities: negative beliefs that prevent us from breaking through. Our expenses will eventually pervade our liabilities over time, as we are only human, and we fall into detrimental patterns unless we condition ourselves. What are your mental and emotional liabilities? Your liabilities encapsulate where you leak; it is where you take away from your potential. What beliefs drain you of your energy, and your ability to cultivate an incredible body? Here are some examples of liabilities: "I believe that if I focus on my body, then I will not be as beautiful on the inside." "I believe that being in shape is just egotistical and unnecessary." "I just do not have the energy to stay in shape." "I am not a healthy person." We must ensure that our assets are stronger than our liabilities.

High Standards

"Set high standards and few limitations for yourself." – Anthony J. D'Angelo

In order to condition ourselves to think, feel and act in ways that will support our physical shape, we must work on our general beliefs first, which will then permeate our beliefs around eating, exercising and health. In life, we must expect the best to happen, yet be prepared for the worst. This way we remain positive and optimistic whilst being prepared to appropriately deal with a difficult circumstance. We must have a strong blueprint as to what we can achieve, and what we expect our current, and future lives, to be like in all aspects: love, finances, hobbies, appearance and so on. Consistent small actions and steps will bring about drastic change. Every day should be even better than the previous. It might just take a small tweak in order to completely implement a new habit that can positively change the course of our direction. Sometimes we may positively change a sequence (thought, emotion and action), but the benefits of this change may not by noticeable until years later. We may think that something lucky just happened to us, but it could have been a direct result of a small change, or many small changes, that we made a long time ago. Think about what happens when striking a golf ball: we come to understand that the most nuanced change in our strike can instigate the most profound change in the course of the golf ball's direction and ultimately where it lands. The same applies to our daily lives: small, useful changes build up incrementally. We can start the transformation now.

We need to trust ourselves. This means ensuring that there is congruency amongst our thoughts, feelings and behaviours. Being aligned and balanced will allow us to truly focus on what we want. It will enable us to get there more quickly and efficiently. Things will work in your favour more if your thoughts, emotions and actions work synchronistically. It is all about creating the right kind of energy both within us and then around us. Someone who is imbalanced in one important area, such as finances, career, relationships and so on, will often be imbalanced in other significant areas. If someone wants to be healthy, yet he or she is emotionally attached to food, then they will have conflicting emotions, and will thus be incongruent within themselves: they are angry and want to change their mind and body, yet they receive instant pleasure and immediate joy when eating addictive foods that are unhealthy. Another example is someone who wants to be wealthy, yet is doing the best he or she can to avoid doing any work, and whose actions tend to be seeking quick get rich schemes, which is almost impossible without studying, discipline and hard work. A third example is someone who wants to get married to a reliable, family-oriented person, yet loves to date exciting, spontaneous people he or she would never settle down with, and so they treat the right person wrongly and the wrong person rightly. It is like completing a puzzle: we need the right pieces in order for everything to fit well together. What we focus on (our thoughts) must coincide with how we feel about its attainment (our attitude), and we must take the necessary actions to make it all happen.

In order to be fully immersed in important experiences, we must condition ourselves to be focused and fully in the moment and even during seemingly innocuous situations. The same applies to the quality of our inner dialogue: we want our inner dialogue to be fully focused on what is happening right in front of us rather than thinking about something totally unrelated. This lack of focus often results in unsupportive thinking, which can negatively affect our health aspirations. We can change this by firstly changing how we are on a smaller scale. For example, if you are watching a film, stay off your phone. If you are having a detailed conversation with someone important to you, remain focused on what they are saying, and not on what you will be doing later. If you are doing work, refrain from having a conversation with someone. If we improve our focus and inner talk during these moments, then we will perform much better when training at the gym or planning our eating schedule and so on because we are fully committed to the immediate experience that is happening right in front of us. The more we can be in the present moment, the more we can make better choices regarding what we eat and how we exercise. It is all about conditioning.

In order to motivate ourselves to consistently make the right choices for our bodies, we must know that we have something that is missing or lacking in our lives. This is often referred to as conscious incompetence. It is not necessarily a bad thing. Feeling that we could improve and do better in the gym or behind the scenes eating is beautiful. People often feel motivated because they feel insufficient. However, it is better to be self-motivated by simply knowing that you have everything you need, but want to give and be even more. Most people would rather keep their hundred pounds (in money) than gain a hundred pounds. The fear of loss is more powerful to most than the pleasure of gaining. If we are to be develop the kind of mind and body we desire, then we must change this mentality. We must make sure that we go for what we really want. Instead of chasing what we can never catch, however, we must have quality habits in place (explored in chapter 10), and simply allow positive things such as mentors, friends and energy etc. to come to us.

When it comes to motivation, we have what is known as toward and away from motivation. Toward motivation is when we want to move closer to something: "I work hard in the gym because I want a six pack." Away from motivation is when we do something in order to move further away from something: "I will not train with people who can help me because I do not want to risk failing and doing poorly in front of them." Interestingly, we can experience both when thinking about the same thing: "I want to train hard at the gym with my peers, but I do not want to be seen as incompetent." This can lead to a lot of frustration, hopelessness and incongruence. We will want to make a choice between whether we want to move closer or further away, and develop affirmations whenever we are thinking about this thing in order to keep us focused (see chapter 10 again). The predominant motivation will soon work its way into our subconscious.

One way of ensuring that we consistently step up and challenge ourselves to be better quality thinkers and doers is to remind ourselves of the kind of commitment, discipline and talent that our role models would portray in our situation. For example, if we are lifting weights, and we are getting closer to failure (not being able to lift anymore), and we think about stopping because it is getting tough, we may benefit from asking ourselves, "What would Ronnie Coleman or Arnold Schwarzenegger do right now?" If we are partaking in a sport, and we are getting tired, then we can ask ourselves: "What would Cristiano Ronaldo do?" or "How would Conor McGregor think in this situation?" We challenge ourselves to think and do what the greats would do, and the same can be applied to our eating habits: "Would Serena Williams eat this way if she was getting ready for a competition?" Compare yourself with the best in certain fields if you want to become incredible in that area.

Goal Setting

"If you don't design your own life plan, chances are you'll fall into someone else's plan. And guess what they have planned for you? Not much." - *Jim Rohn*

We must know where we want to go in life otherwise we will fall into mediocrity as it relates to our bodies and health. If we do not know where we are heading, then how will we get there? How will we know if we are on track? We could spend all our time labouring and gathering resources for the journey, but if the destination is right next to us then what was the point? We must write out our long-term goals (such as to lose 15lbs of fat), and break them down into small, simple and actionable steps that make our quality goals appear more easily surmountable. What will you need to learn to get the body you want? What will you need to buy regularly to maintain your quality eating habits? What kind of support mechanisms will you need around you to keep you on track?

It is absolutely crucial to set goals for ourselves (short-term, medium-term and long-term goals) because they will keep us focused and disciplined. We live in a world where we are bombarded with so much information that it is hard to stay focused on absolutely anything for a sustained period of time, let alone something every day. We are so accustomed to incessantly checking our phones, and having our immediate attention taken by various marketing tools, that we can get lost in a world of other people's wants, and, thus, we lose focus on the things that we want! It is so easy to get sidetracked, and to fall off the bandwagon of health. We need to have a result in mind; most importantly we need to know *why* we want to achieve something, and we need an action plan to ensure that we get it for a specific date.

"A goal is a dream with a deadline." - Napoleon Hill

We are more likely to achieve what we want if we focus on it and remain driven. We want to make it habitual. We will want to write out your goals daily or at the very least weekly. Be as specific as possible when setting goals. What makes a goal more powerful? Firstly, we can phrase it positively by using the robust modal verb, 'will.' For example, "I will lose 15lbs of fat." Secondly, we must outline the specific things that we want. For example, "I will lose 15lbs of fat, so that I can have the kind of energy I want to thrive, and so that I can feel confident enough to attract the kind of partner I want." Thirdly, we have to set a deadline for this goal, which makes us more accountable as we know things will have to happen (taking action in different ways) for us to achieve this goal. For example, "I will lose 15lbs of fat by August 1st, so that I can have the kind of energy I want to thrive, and so that I can feel confident enough to attract the kind of partner I want." It can be even more powerful to phrase this as though it is already happening. Assuming that we already have what we want can subconsciously trick our minds into thinking that it is already there. We attract what we truly believe in.

We should always have at least three important goals in our lives. It could be our health, relationships and wealth for example. Even though these key areas seem unrelated, you will notice that the more you succeed in one area, the more momentum and energy you generate, which can support you in the other two areas. What do we do every day to help transform these wishes into our reality? We should remind ourselves of our goals each day, and feel grateful for the opportunity to pursue them without having to endure crippling circumstances. Little things combined result in the accomplishment of monumental things. What ways of thinking and actions can we introduce today to achieve our goals, desires and dreams? What can we do today to bring ourselves a step closer to this vision? Whom could we converse with to inspire or provide essential knowledge? What could we research? What seminars could we attend? Why not sign up to it today? What books, from people who have achieved in this field, could we read? Who are our role models in this field? How can we learn about their aptitudes and experiences as a way of motivating and modelling?

If we are not improving something, then its strength will subside day by day. Routines that are outdated need to be reexamined. What was once passionate can be passionate again. If we want to, or need to, improve our health, then what could we do today to support our energy and longevity? The Internet provides great copious information as it relates to health and fitness. What grocery stores do you go to? What is your standard shopping list? What is stored inside your fridge? How active are you every week? Sometimes we just need to stop reflecting and just do. Nothing is holding us back.

We do not need all of the latest gym equipment or health shakes. All we need to do is invest in our health in order to do what is necessary. We should invest our time, energy and resources into our health. Without our health, everything else is meaningless and can capitulate as a result.

Always have another goal in place, which you are already working towards, just before you achieve your original goal in order to sustain your drive. For example, if your goal is to lose 15lbs of fat, then you can also be working on your next goal of gaining 15lbs of muscle. It keeps your momentum going once you have accomplished your original goal. This does not mean you should not celebrate where you are now; just have the motions set in place for the next step. You should always be content and happy with where you are, but it is highly beneficial to know your next endeavour. Move towards your blueprint with intensity, and refuse to allow anything to compromise its cultivation.

Everything in life is connected. Our lifestyle is a reflection of our beliefs. Our lifestyle determines our path: if we eat garbage, see our friends for too long, do too many things that are urgent but unimportant, then it is clear that it will take us a long time to accomplish a goal let alone many goals. If we want to accelerate the process, then we must become more productive, judicious and disciplined every single day. Whatever we think about manifests into our lives (but only if action is taken). We find what we look for. Unfortunately, people have conditioned themselves to either look for the wrong things or wander around looking for anything. Have you ever bought a car, and then all of a sudden you saw that car seemingly everywhere? We attract what we focus on. Therefore, we must do our utmost to remain focused on things that support us. Those who wander and meander through life are the ones who fall into other people's plans; they are the ones who get sidetracked, caught up in petty squabbles and drama. Good things may show up, but will we be opportunistic enough to take advantage of them? Will we react flexibly, and with clarity in thought and movement? There are openings and opportunities around us every day to help us better ourselves, but we must have the mental clarity to conceive them.

Visualisation

"A picture is worth a thousand words." – Napoleon

Visualisation can be a magnificent tool. Some people say they are not creative, but this just means that they have limiting beliefs regarding their imagination. We have to be able to imagine getting what we want. If we can visualise things in our minds, then they can be manifested into reality. One must be able to visualise, and believe in the possibility of such a thing coming true. Without conceiving the possibility, our thoughts, feeling and actions will never work congruently to achieve our desires. NLP (Neuro-linguistic programming) cofounders, Richard Bandler and John Grinder, teach how to visualise in the most potent of ways, so please look into their work. Some sub-modalities of visualisation involve making the picture we want to materialise brighter and clearer, viewing it as though it is right in front of us (seen through our eyes) with movement and sound as opposed to seeing it within a 'frame' like the kind of frame around a portrait.

These strong sub-modalities will serve to motivate us further, as the mind finds it hard to distinguish between what is real and what is imagined. If you imagine it vividly enough, and often enough, then the mind will act as though it is already here, and so we will act in ways that will naturally create such beautiful things. We must be able to imagine its possibility, and use the techniques of NLP along with incantations to drive it into the unconscious. However, to materialise this desire, we must follow our intuition, and take action quickly rather than delaying or hesitating. The ability to imagine oneself being successful at something is crucial. It can be challenging to distinguish dreams from reality at times; therefore, being able to imagine success signals to the brain that it can be achieved. The brain is unable to distinguish the difference between something that is visually constructed and that which is a real visual moment. We can, therefore, use this to our advantage by playing them out more favourably in our minds. Nothing exists in reality unless it was once imagined. Life has a very interesting way of bringing things into our lives if we know exactly what it is we want, and, of course, if we take massive pertinent action.

"Imagination is more important than knowledge." – Albert Einstein

Imagination can be more profound than knowledge as it relates to bringing our goals into realisation. Our imagination holds incredible power, yet many people do not take the time to visualise what they want in their lives. They fail to coerce their own mind into conceiving a promising future. Why? It is deemed unconventional, outlandish and thus weird. I do not know about you, but I would rather be bizarre and happy rather than normal and depressed. This visual impetus can help in creating a shift; it creates the possibility of a compelling future, and gives us the motivation to take pertinent actions to manifest the life we want. Visualisation and affirmations alone will not magically gift us the life that we want. However, it can begin to set positive outcomes in motion. Visualisation develops the confidence required to continue taking action even when things might not be going according to plan, or if things still seem so far away. As William Blake once proclaimed, "What is now proved was once only imagined." Therefore, we may never have the life we want if we have never imagined its possibility in meticulous, vivid detail. We can only create what we can imagine. We give life to what we imagine. Moreover, what we think about before and after sleep is pivotal as these ideas accentuate and perpetuate our beliefs. What we read, study or visualise before and after sleep become more deeply embedded within our long-term memory and subconscious.

"What is now proved was once only imagined." –
William Blake

Pleasure and Pain

"The secret of success is learning how to use pain and pleasure instead of having pain and pleasure use you. If you do that, you're in control of your life. If you don't, life controls you." – Tony Robbins

Our psychology, associations and beliefs dictate the course of our lives. Consider whether you associate more pleasure or pain to the following situations: Do you feel more pleasure or pain when eating an unhealthy dessert? What about once you have finished eating it? Do you feel more pleasure or pain when you go to the gym? What about once you are finished? Do you feel more pleasure or pain by waking up early in the morning to get hard work done? Everyone will have different answers especially before and during these activities, but more people will agree that they feel much better after they did the challenging activities. This is the key to succeeding in life. It is not about enjoying things before or during all of the time. It is about how you will feel once you have stepped up and completed the activity.

Really the pleasure and pain principle is all about how we frame things to ourselves. We can easily change these perceptions if we generate enough leverage. For instance, if we said that there is more pleasure in eating an unhealthy dessert than pain, then we can easily manipulate this evaluation. We just need to find something more powerful than our current associations: eating too many of these foods can make us obese, suffer from illnesses, die earlier, and, thus, limit the time we have with our family and friends in this realm; eating too many of these foods can stop us from attracting the kind of partner we really want, or make us struggle to keep him or her for that matter; eating too many of these foods can show how mentally and emotionally weak we are. If we use certain trigger words to anger us, then we can stop ourselves from falling into any of these negative choices. If we weigh things up, by thinking longer term, we will be able to generate enough leverage to change our pleasure and pain beliefs.

We cannot manifest anything into our lives if our thoughts and belief systems are incongruent or contradictory. For example, if we want the sexiest husband, but we are afraid of being cheated on, then these beliefs are in opposition, and so the mind will either release the cultivation of its manifestation altogether, or move toward the thought with the most emotion tied to it. So if we are more afraid of the possibility of their impending infidelity, more than our love for a gorgeous counterpart, then we may live a life single or not getting what we really want. If we want to start a successful business, but we also want to live a relaxed lifestyle, then these two forces oppose, and so you end up in the middle or with neither. No outcome is worse, but only different, and it is a choice. The same applies to our physical body: if we want an amazing body, but we want to go out drinking and eating what we feel like having, then we obviously have conflicting desires. This will lead to great internal conflict and pain until we choose one once and for all.

Emotional Trauma

"Someone who has experienced trauma also has gifts to offer all of us – in their depth, their knowledge of our universal vulnerability, and their experience of the power of compassion." –
Sharon Salzberg

One of the things that inhibit our ability to develop the kind of mind and body we really want is the trauma we may have sustained at some point in our past. Whether we like to admit it or not, obesity is a direct result of some form of emotional struggle. In order to allow ourselves to become obese, there must be some level of emotional pain involved otherwise people would not compromise their health and wellbeing to such degree. It is oftentimes a reflection of not having enough stability and balance. Obesity is often a sign of negligence in one form or another. It demonstrates either some form of trauma, or how the individual has either been let down, or how they perceive themselves to have been let down by someone or something. Overweight people are trying to fill some sort of emotional hole. The body is a reflection of the mind. Obese individuals are clearly addicted to something. They may be addicted to sugar or overeating, and so this must be traced back to the root of the problem. What has caused this kind of irresponsible and careless behaviour? Once we find out what has traumatised the individual, then we can address the problem.

What are examples of possible trauma? Obese individuals may feel as though their parents never accepted them, and so they feel like they are not enough as they are, and so they overcompensate by eating. Obese individuals may have been emotionally or physically abused, and so they turn to food as a source of joy and appeasement. Obese individuals may feel helpless as a result of losing someone they loved, and so they have essentially given up caring about themselves; they have lost their self-esteem and their pride has been broken. Additionally, they may be overworking, trying to prove themselves, and have suppressed their inner desires. Obese individuals have not yet been able to find more supportive ways of dealing with stress.

If we do not address the current, or past, issues in our lives, then we may be able to lose a few pounds of fat, but this weight will often find its way back home because we have not dealt with its key emotional triggers. Even having an insufficient blueprint can be a sign of low self-esteem, as mentally healthy individuals always want to improve in life's key areas, which partly consist of our health and physical body. Unhealthy individuals can become healthy if they are self-reflective and honest with themselves. However, people with large egos will refuse to admit that they have some form of emotional shortcomings. Clarity is power. We must dig deep into our psychology if we are to rewire the interchanges between our thoughts, emotions and actions.

Chapter 2: Psychology – Invest

"Personal development is the belief that you are worth the effort, time and energy needed to develop yourself." - Denis Waitley

The more we invest our time, energy and money into our health and physical shape, the more we value our health and physical shape. We are attaching our thoughts and feelings to it to such degree that we feel deeply connected, and so are less inclined to give up or place other things ahead of it. We value what we invest in. For example, imagine that you wanted to go on a renowned fat-loss course. Consider two scenarios that outline the different things experienced, but for the exact same tickets. Scenario 1: Your friends bought you the tickets at a reduced price; the event will be local to where you live, and the event will take place during a quiet weekend for you. Scenario 2: You had to research long and hard to find the tickets, and they cost a bomb! The event will take place in a neighbouring city, and the event, unfortunately, is scheduled for a weekend where you also have other obligations. Let us say that you hypothetically went to the event for both scenarios. You will definitely be more committed to the material presented in the course if you experienced scenario 2 rather than scenario 1. This would be the case for all of us. Why? Because you sacrificed more to attend the event where you invested more time (researching the tickets and travelling to the event), more energy (researching, driving, rescheduling the weekend's activities etc.) and more money (paying a high price for the tickets and travels).

This is why it is crucial for us to invest our time, energy and money into our mental and physical health. This can be done in many ways. For example, we can invest our time developing our physical shape by researching nutritional aspects or exercise regimes, or we can become qualified within these areas and teach others (all forms of investing time in our bodies). Moreover, we can invest our energy by attending gym classes or travelling to our gym consistently (even for something small such as going into a sauna and so on). Additionally, we can invest our money by paying a personal trainer for one-to-one sessions, or paying for quality nutritional foods and supplements, or even paying to get professional pictures taken of ourselves. Consider the ways in which you invest in these three avenues, as it relates to your health, fitness and physique. Are you investing enough? Why must we continue to invest in our health?

We now need to act as though we already have this dream body. We will need to only buy outfits that our ideal selves will fit into well. This is massively important because we are not only committing to this transformation, but we are teaching our subconscious that this is the way things need to be from now on, and we have to adapt to it. We also need to change our behaviours to match this new and improved physique. How would someone act and behave if they had this new body? Surely, we would be more confident with our appearance, and our ability to make what was once impossible now possible. Surely our new selves deserve to either attract a better quality partner if single, or receive the kind of physical attention required from our existing partners. We need to act as though we are this way now, even if we are not there yet. We are teaching the brain to perceive anew.

Suffer and Succeed

"Suffer now and live the rest of your life as a champion." – Muhammad Ali

Nothing will change unless a person has suffered enough. The harder we work for something, the more we appreciate it. The more time we invest in helping our siblings, the more we love them, and want to give them (especially if it is appreciated). The more money we spend on healthy products and services, the more we value our health. The more energy we give our partners, the more we value them. Consider your life patterns. Think about how much time, money and energy we give to feeding awful habits, and think about how little we give to areas in our lives that are actually important. The more we struggle and give now, the better our futures will be. The more comfortable we feel in the uncomfortable, the more successful we shall be. Nothing is meaningful, valuable and desirable unless we have invested sufficient energy and time into it. We must work hard at something to feel a true sense of accomplishment. Without hardship, adversity, persistence, challenge and so on, we will not exhibit lasting change. These feelings do not derive from inheriting things, pure luck or charity of some sort. We only truly appreciate something if we fought and thought for its attainment.

There is a balance to everything: the more we struggle for something, the more we will be rewarded by it. If we suffer for something now, then we will experience great happiness in the future. However, we must be tenacious enough to stick with it. People often give up right before they would have begun to see results. If we have been heartbroken and devastated, a beautiful and loving relationship is on the horizon. If we exercise and expend a great deal of energy, we will later be exhausted yet fulfilled. If we train intensely and suffer physically, our muscles will develop. Our muscles expand due to intense demand and excruciating pain. The harder we work for something, the more rewarding it shall be. Conquer challenges and build momentum in everything we believe to be worthwhile. Short-term discomfort leads to long-term happiness. Inertia leads to long-term affliction.

Success, as it relates to our minds, bodies, relationships, finances, careers and so on, requires a great deal of affliction. If the road to marriage was too easy, then the road to divorce would be just as easy. There is no need to unnecessarily create barriers or challenges, but we must work on what we want! We must invest in our relationships. People get married, and then they take their foot off the pedal. They stop working on themselves. They stop supporting each other. They believe they have accomplished what they set out to do. Wrong. If we are not learning or investing our energy into any important relationship (with people or priorities), then it is slowly deteriorating. If we think that our partners are just going to live contently the way he or she is now, then we are wrong. If it is not progressing, it is declining, and we will suffer greatly as a result. Incidentally, one of the reasons why a significantly high percentage of lottery winners lose their entire winnings is because they did not earn it. It was given to them. They neither appreciate it the same way, nor do they know what to do with it. Why? They never invested substantial time, money and energy into its cultivation.

The more we suffer for something, the more we learn to love it. The more energy we invest in something, the more we value it. This is why it is necessary to suffer for our children; this is the problem with many wealthy families who delegate all parental responsibilities to a nanny for instance. There will inevitably be a disconnection between parent and child. Why do we think childbirth is so painful? Think about the things we suffer for, and consider if we value these things more than other things that just happen easily for us. If we are spoilt as a child, we do not grow up to value money. If we are used to winning all the time, then we do not learn and grow from these experiences. If we do not struggle for the physical body we want, then we will not experience the bliss of our struggles. Earn it; enjoy it.

Love to Learn

"Every moment of one's existence, one is growing into more or retreating into less." - **Norman Mailer**

A love of learning is invaluable. It fills our lives with great joy, as we feel like we are constantly becoming better and thus happier. It serves to massively reduce moments of boredom and sadness whilst keeping our brains active and challenged, which is even more useful as we age. If we love to learn, then we can always occupy our minds when alone or bored. There is always something to do; there is always something interesting to learn. It is a healthy mindset that keeps us away from negative, decadent habits. Nonetheless, we should choose to learn about topics that are important, and not just learning for the sake of learning. We should research and study what interests us. It is always beneficial to research and explore key fundamental areas such as how relationships work (communication, rapport and psychology), health (what fuels us and supports the brain's function) and wealth (forms of active and passive income). This ensures that we remain balanced and in control of our lives, which will indirectly positively affect your physical shape.

Learning any new skill, or new information, can be easier if we have the right mindset. We can learn and develop more quickly if we approach the activity as though it is a simple concept or skill to acquire. Some people may think, "I am about to learn something new, but it takes me ages to learn new things." What we say about ourselves, whether they are supportive or not, will become our reality. We should never say that we cannot do something because that is the narrative we paint for ourselves; we build walls around us that prevent us from learning and thus growing. The phrase, "takes me ages," sets in stone exactly how we absorb meaning. Furthermore, some people say things like, "I could never be a doctor," or "I am just not physically coordinated." We must take the words "I can't" out of our vocabulary. What we believe in becomes our reality. Additionally, we must ensure that we are in the right state to learn: sit upright, be positive and optimistic, and focus on the present moment. Moreover, we must remove any clutter in the mind; the clearer our thoughts, the easier it is to literally store and retain information in our long-term memory.

In addition, we must ensure that we act upon the material we have just learnt. We will need to make changes quickly after we have learned this new information. We can take what we have just learned, and kinesthetically and physically do something to embed this new information. Start the momentum. See if we can apply this newfound knowledge within different contexts. See if we can make connections between topics and skills that we know very well, and whatever it is that is now being learnt. Moreover, we can make some kind of personal or emotional connection with the material we are learning in order to ensure that it stays within our long-term memory. Unfortunately, many people hear or see something interesting, yet they then communicate something to themselves along the lines of, "I'll get to that soon," or "it's great that I've learnt that" (without even putting it into practice yet), or "I should definitely try this one day." The problem with these phrases is that they create distance between their new thoughts and delayed actions. They have logically understood that something is great and beneficial, but they leave it so long that their emotions have not been engaged deeply enough, and thus no action will follow suit down the line. This is why we would benefit from taking the material within this book, and embed them within ourselves as soon as possible otherwise this will only be an interesting book and nothing more profound for us. We think, feel and listen to so much information every single day that it is hard to simply pluck things out and embed them in our minds permanently. This freshly instilled knowledge (and subsequent action) must be exercised frequently to ensure that enough energy and emotion has been invested into its worth. The more we revisit information, the more it becomes embedded into our long-term memory.

We must know who we are, what we are like, and how we function if we are to create the kind of physical body we want. This level of meta-cognition and self-comprehension is crucial. Understanding what we like, what we dislike and how we filter information allows us to be more efficient with our time. If we know how we learn best, then we most efficiently learn this new material: what space do you learn best in? Do you like to study independently? Do you prefer discussing key topics around health and fat loss with friends etc.? When at work, how do you perform at your best? In terms of your relationship, what mindset enables you to get the most out of yourself? Having an honest and loving relationship with ourselves will help us to learn information better. If we learn information better, then we develop better self-esteem. If we have strong self-esteem then we take care of ourselves better: we stop smoking, drinking excessively, we ensure that we sleep better, we keep hydrated, we choose highly nutritious earth-grown foods more often and so on. Our self-esteem is very much connected to our mental health and thus our physical health.

We should take the time to learn from our experiences and from the experiences of others. We must value learning and developing otherwise the apathy and indifference accumulated over time will come back to us in harsher and more painful ways. A painful experience is a chance to reflect and learn. By not reflecting and learning a valuable lesson, then the same lesson will come back twofold. This 'compound pain' repeats itself until we break the habit, and attack the source of the problem: usually us. If we think about it, everything compounds. Just like compound interest in monetary terms, we invest something (our money for instance), and then we reinvest again whilst keeping the original sum. This is why people get more devastated every time they incur a meaningful setback. Their affliction compounds. The same works in the positive realm. Invest time and energy into the creation of something beautiful such as our health and physical shape, and then our next creation (getting more muscular or lean for example) will have the success from the previous one along with whatever new skill we have now developed. This is oftentimes why most people fail with their first 'business' venture or diet. If they continue to learn and attempt new businesses or diets, then they will learn more lessons and eventually succeed. If we want a better body, then we cannot give up or assume that we have tried everything. Our mentality determines our physical shape over time. We must learn from our previous errors, and accumulated massive strengths, lessons and resources to support us when we come back to the same issue: fat loss, lean muscle development etc.

Our Surroundings

"Surround yourself with only people who are going to lift you higher."
– Oprah Winfrey

We also invest in our friends, family, colleagues and so on. We invest in people when we listen to them and spend time with them. These interactions either directly or indirectly have some kind of effect on our physical shape. Whom do we surround ourselves with? We must have positive role models around us if we are to have the kind of energy needed to keep moving forward, and to make better decisions regarding our health. We tend to develop similar habits as our friends. If they eat unhealthily, then we are more likely to eat unhealthily. If they drink and smoke, then we are more likely to drink or smoke. If our friends are wasteful with their time, then we will be more wasteful with ours, and we have already explored how our self-esteem is tied to our physical bodies.

We must surround ourselves with people who have high standards for their health and bodies. They say that your finances are the average of your five closest friends. I also believe this applies to our health and bodies. Obviously friends usually go out together, and we learn each other's eating patterns just like we learn each other's sayings. If we have obese friends, then we can still stay in contact with them, but it would be ideal not to be around them too much or too often. The more rapport we have with our friends, the more we are likely to take on their thoughts, emotions and actions. Be mindful of this.

"There is nothing noble in being superior to your fellow man; true nobility is being superior to your former self." - Ernest Hemingway

We must also consider the strengths and talents within our friendship groups. Are you more intelligent than your friends when it comes to nutrition, exercise and fitness? Are you healthier than your friends? Are you more accomplished, mentally, physically or financially than your friends? If the answer is yes, then you are letting yourself down dreadfully. We must ensure that we are stimulated, challenged and continuously progressing by spending time with other highly successful, healthy and motivated people. If we are stronger than our peers in areas of great importance, then we are letting our egos get the better of us. Weaker people like spending time with people they feel more successful than. This is detrimental. We must always learn and grow if we are to maximise our potential. It is not about being better than others; it is about being our best possible selves. We must be mindful of what we listen to regularly. We will adopt many of the beliefs and thought patterns of those we are closest to, so we must be selective with whom we spend our time with, and how often we spend time with them.

Moreover, the actual noise, words and loudness of what we hear can influence us greatly. Think about what we hear every single day. Who is it coming from, and in what form is it coming from? We must ensure that we listen to positive, enriching people otherwise we will fall into mediocre and unsuccessful patterns. Also, we must be conscious of the type of music that we listen to, as aggressive music can make us more aggressive, and depressing music can make us feel sadder and so on. Whilst playing with our emotions enables us to experience emotional variety, we must be cautious of the emotions we allow ourselves to experience each day. If they become addictive, then we search for them in other contexts. Human beings naturally want to create more, but we also have a tendency of wanting to get more of what we already have and that includes the thoughts and experiences we see and hear. For example, people who watch dramatic television and reality shows tend to behave in ways that emulate some of these situations whether wittingly or unwittingly. It may sound daft, but it is the truth. We move toward what we see. We move toward what we listen to and accept.

In terms of our physical surroundings, we must ensure that our bedrooms, flats or houses are consistently clean. Our physical surroundings are a direct reflection of our minds. If writing or computer-based work is a priority, then ensure that your desk is clear and only equipped with essential stationery. If your family keeps you motivated, then have a picture of them in front of you when working, so that you turn to them in moment of challenge. The same applies to religious imagery or religious quotations, and having pictures of our role models around us. We want our settings to give us the clarity and strength needed because these are the physical places where we shape our lives. Wherever you write your goals, study or read, make sure that the surrounding area is clean and organised. It would have pictures of your physical role models around you in order to keep you focused, and that you set high standards for yourself. Seeing or hearing from these influential people remind us of their talents and what we want for ourselves.

We must focus on the positives. We must refrain from giving energy to things that are harmful. For example, if there is a colossal car accident on the motorway, then purposely choose not to look at it as you drive by because it is important not to focus on negative things. Additionally, purposely avoid the news primarily because it focuses on sad, negative things; we search for the things we see and experience most often. Avoid spending time with dramatic people, or people who are severely unlucky chiefly because we wish to experience positive, supportive things. We will attract wonderful things because we are loving, giving and friendly. Know, deep down, that we deserve success, and we deserve to have the body we want. We must see the wider picture, and act based upon positive thoughts and emotions: thoughts are more accurate and clear by its very nature whereas emotions are thoughts that are unquantifiable and indefinable. Thought occurs when we are proactive, and emotion occurs when we are reactive. The better we plan and preempt things from happening, the more in control we will feel as it relates to our healthy eating and exercise schedules.

Knowledge is not power. Knowledge that is executed is power. Most of us know roughly what we should eat, and what types of exercise we should implement, but our shoulds will never get done because they are clearly not a priority for us. Whatever is a must for us will be carried out. Our health and self-esteem are some of the most important things to anyone in life. They must be. We cannot take them for granted because we are either improving or getting worse. If we take things for granted, such as our health and being in average shape, then we will make unnecessary mistakes down the line. It is about taking responsibility, and doing what is right. It is not selfish to take care of your health, your appearance and how you feel. It is selfish to not model by example, so that you can positively influence hundreds if not thousands of people you interact with in life.

Modelling

"We like to think of our champions and idols as superheroes who were born different from us. We don't like to think of them as relatively ordinary people who made themselves extraordinary." - Carol S. Dweck

A large part of mastering our health and physical shape is to learn from the most successful and talented people within these areas. All we need to do is emulate their beliefs, thought patterns and emotions (to a certain extent). We should pay attention to the way in which they carry themselves, the way they dress, how they speak about health, fat loss and muscle gain and what their general beliefs are as many of our beliefs can be linked to health in one way or another. The more we adopt from these brilliant individuals, the more likely we are to attract some of their qualities. We begin to think and act more like them, and so we can attract the kind of great things that they attract. Naturally people can only become masters within one or two fields (as it takes such dedication, effort and experience), but by studying them meticulously, we can also master, or come close to mastering, what they have done by simply taking on their perceptions and the things that they do successfully. Ultimately, it is always better to be yourself, but there is nothing wrong with incorporating the qualities of some of the most successful people in the world. There is nothing wrong with exaggerating your current features, so that you become more like the strong, successful men and/or women that you appreciate.

These role models do not have to specialise directly in health, fat loss and muscle gain. We can also notice many very important principles from those who are masters in seemingly unrelated fields. For example, Warren Buffett teaches the importance of staying within your own circle of competence as a way of becoming wealthy. We can adopt the same principle and apply it to fat loss/muscle gain: we must know what foods and dietary strategies work well for us, and primarily stick to these as our long-term strategies for health. Additionally, Steve Jobs used to dress the same way daily in order to make life simpler. We can do the same by choosing similar meals to have on most days for example. We can also choose to wear certain, convenient things, and to look a certain way, so they we free up more time in the mornings to fit in our workouts etc. Think about the people you admire, regardless of what fields they are in, and contemplate their biggest strengths. See if you can link some of their beliefs and strategies to the world of health and fitness.

We can consistently feed our brains inspirational and encouraging stories about all positive things that can somehow relate to fat loss and great health. We move toward what we focus on. Unfortunately, many people gravitate to negative stories or stories about people who had it all and lost it (because it supports the story in their minds that you cannot always progress). Instead, we can inundate ourselves with successful stories and transformational information, so that we can continue to grow. Obviously, learning from our role models' psychology and mechanics can be highly beneficial, but be more interested in their psychology (how they perceive things) rather than their mechanics (the things they actually do). What mindset and experiences led to their greatness? How do they think, and what do they do in terms of activities? What are their daily routines? What do they avoid doing? What were the key moments in their lives and why? Analyse and adopt the vocabulary they use. Here are some examples of stars who have been able to transform their physical bodies, which is then followed by example of stars who have had amazing bodies and health for decades.

Some stars who have lost weight considerably:

Jennifer Hudson

"When you're shopping you forget about eating!"
- Jennifer Hudson

Musical artist, Jennifer Hudson, is not only massively talented vocally, but she also managed to totally transform her body after American Idol. Interestingly, she did not do so by exercising much. Instead she completely dedicated herself to eating healthily. Consciously, she now only eats foods that fuel her. No one can argue with the results. Whilst her quotation is fittingly funny, it totally relates to the penultimate chapter in this book: Keep Busy and Active. Once you get all the variety you need in one avenue (shopping for example), then you do not need that level of variety elsewhere (such as with food). Consider the ways in which you get variety and excitement in your life. If food falls into that category, then simply think of other ways you can achieve variety and uncertainty as a way of making life feel more liberating and diverse.

Melissa McCarthy

"I have a real obsession with people who just do not care." - Melissa McCarthy

Due to her great fame, Melissa unfairly received scrutiny for her physical size, and she was only getting cast in certain roles. Controversially, Melissa claims that she started to lose substantial weight due to a fat loss supplement: Garcinia Cambogia. Relentlessly, Melissa was criticised for the way in which she claimed to have lost weight, and she also lost her role in *Mike and Molly,* as she did not look the part anymore apparently. Pleasingly, Melissa is rightly more excited about her physical transformation more than her roles as an actress. Good for her. We can also learn that we will never make everybody happy regardless of how much we positively change our physical shape. The way we feel about ourselves is more important. Moreover, we should also put our health and dream bodies ahead of our careers. Always put health above wealth even though they are inherently linked in many ways.

Jonah Hill

"You really feel an obligation to someone when they're trusting you to do something, and you promise that you'll come through for them." –
Jonah Hill

Think about the people who are closest to you. Make a promise to them that you will lose a certain amount of weight by a certain time. Tell them to hold you accountable. When you publicise your intentions, you become responsible, and we do not want to disappoint those who are closest to us. Not only will you benefit tremendously, but also your physical and mental improvements will inspire those around you. Do it for yourself, but more importantly, do it for others. The more we give, the more we wish to produce. Jonah, having been overweight for so long, which suited the roles he played in movies up until now, clearly lost weight quite significantly. He claims that he did this by hiring a nutritionist, and he started to use a food journal to monitor his eating habits. Whilst he seems to have added some muscle to his physique, it is obvious that Jonah values the importance of eating quality food, as it is far more important than how much we exercise. As a percentage, nutrition should be seen as contributing to overall fat loss by 75% whereas our exercise and training equate to just 25%.

Some stars who have consistently incredible bodies:

Dwayne Johnson

"Once you've ever been hungry, really, really hungry, then you'll never, ever be full." - Dwayne Johnson

The 'Rock' usually begins his day training at four o'clock in the morning. He starts with his cardio, and then has his breakfast. Subsequently, he would go to the gym to lift weights, and then he would go to work. He works out twice before the average human being wakes up. Interestingly, he likes to workout twice before he goes to work because he feels like he can spend the rest of the day working, and still feel satisfied that he did his training that day. He averages around five hours of sleep. We must take Dwayne's huge physical frame into consideration, but he eats between six to seven meals per day.

Intelligently, he hires a strength and conditioning coach and a dietary coach even though he knows a lot about training and nutrition! His eating schedule consists of mostly lean meats, fish, egg whites and greens. We must always look to make our workouts more challenging whether it is by lifting heavier weights, doing more reps or sets, or resting less between sets.

Arnold Schwarzenegger

"Just like in bodybuilding, failure is also a necessary experience for growth in our own lives, for if we're never tested to our limits, how will we know how strong we really are? How will we ever grow?" - Arnold Schwarzenegger

Arnold advocates that we must burn more calories than we eat if we are to lose weight. Additionally, he states that we must do at least two hundred crunches every single day. He claims doing the 'vacuum,' which is essentially all about pulling our stomachs in as much as possible and holding it there for fifteen seconds for at least three reps. He asserts that it teaches the mind to subconsciously pull the stomach in, so that our stomachs shrink and stay small. Moreover, Arnold foregrounds the importance of keeping our postures and bodies straight generally; he also believes this is necessary when performing our exercises. Furthermore, Arnold often talks about training with people who were even better than him at certain key exercises, such as squats, as a way of making him perform his own squats better. We must be able to put our egos aside if we are to learn from others. He advocates doing no more than three sets per body part for beginners because he knows the dangers of overtraining especially what overtraining can do to people who give things up quite quickly. Once we begin to develop certain body parts better than others, then Arnold advocates doing more sets for weaker body parts in order to make the body more proportionate.

Jennifer Lopez

"I love the way working out makes me feel, so I try to keep my body hydrated and well rested after every workout." – Jennifer Lopez

Jenifer Lopez believes that there is not one ideal. There are no magic secrets. It is simple: not too much partying, sleep well and train often. You have to care about yourself, and take care of yourself. Unsurprisingly, Jennifer starts her day off with a protein shake in the morning. Then she has some fruit before lunch or a health bar. Subsequently, Jennifer has chicken and salad and quinoa. Amusingly, she prefers to add lemon to many foods in order to make it taste sweeter whilst providing the alkalizing benefits that lemons provide. Moreover, she asserts that it is all about portion control. She advocates everything in moderation. It is not good to totally deprive yourself. Passionately, JLO explains that we must always think about what we want to accomplish. Have short-term goals in mind to excite us, and motivate us to remain focused. Then you get into a good routine, and getting compliments helps to keep us motivated, which will happen naturally if we keep losing fat. This is all about momentum and ensuring that we reward ourselves for doing well consistently. JLo has tried all kinds of diets etc., but every person is different. Some things may work for men whereas other supplements are geared towards women, so it is really about knowing how our bodies work and what is good for us.

Chapter 3: Psychology – Negativity, the Ego and Food

If we are to understand our current physical situation, then we must explore how our thoughts, emotions and actions are interconnected. Also, we must comprehend how the mind works, so that we can consistently make better choices, and thus create the ideal body we want to maintain. The mind and body are closely connected. We must continuously look after one, so that the other can benefit: when we look after our minds, then we look after our bodies, and when we look after our bodies, then we take care of our minds. Moreover, we will look at the ego, its purpose, and the many different forms of fear (stemming from the ego) that often ruin our chances of developing the bodies we want and deserve.

Thoughts, Emotions and Actions

"Human behavior flows from three main sources: desire, emotion, and knowledge." - Plato

Not all thoughts turn into actions. Only thoughts that have enough emotion attached to them turn into physical actions. So what are thoughts? Thoughts are very direct and clear statements. What are emotions then? Emotions can be seen as thoughts that are unclear, ambiguous, indiscernible, and thus are more gripping. The more we break an emotion down in terms of what has caused it, the looser its grip becomes. These emotions (unclear thoughts) are either negative or positive. So, for example, if you have a thought that says, "I could get into the best shape of my life," and if you have a strong emotion (say excitement or intrigue) that attaches itself to this thought, then you will take some kind of action and press forward (say write a plan of action for yourself, or talk to someone who can support you and so on). Unfortunately, there are two sides to the coin. Another thought could be, "I'm just not mentally strong enough," and if this thought creates a strong emotion within you (such as sadness or hopelessness), which you entertain, then you will act in a way that conforms to this judgement: you may detach yourself from others, or blame someone when the topic is brought up, or you may just become inert and indolent. We want to remain indifferent to unsupportive thoughts. Let them pass by.

Being analytical and evaluative are great skills, but over-thinking can be perilous. Why? Because when we over-think, the negative voice (which exists within us all) tends to show up more as over-thinking frequently creates uncertainty. Subsequently, our imagination takes over, and we begin to play out all of the different possibilities in our minds, which further complicates matters, often resulting in disempowering outcomes. Thoughts and emotions have different energy; emotions clearly contain much more energy than pure thoughts. This is why incantations (covered in chapter 10) add power and substance to our thoughts (as motion creates emotion and vice versa).

What makes a thought spring to mind? Past conditioning, associations, primitive desires (id), our understanding of right from wrong, our values (superego) and so on. A thought consists of the language we have accrued being formed syntactically to make sense and to direct understanding. The words we learn and know are so significant. If you want to have a better body and health, then predominantly speak of quality, positive things with rich vocabulary. How would you describe your current physique for instance? If you want to be leaner and healthier, then study the terms and vocabulary that the shredded and healthy learn and use. Conversely, understand the words that the obese and unhealthy use especially around nutrition and exercise, and steer away from their lexis. In a way, we must exaggerate things to ourselves in order to motivate and influence ourselves. For instance, if you wake up, and you think that, "Today is just going to be another monotonous, average day," then how badly do you want to jump out of bed and get on with it? Alternatively, if you wake up, and think, "I am going to kill it today. It is going to be a massively important day, and I am going to give it my all," then I am sure you will get out of bed with more zest!

Intriguingly, in the brilliant book, *Emotional Intelligence*, Daniel Goleman explores LeDeoux's research, which expresses the human brain's evolutionary process. Our brains have developed tremendously, and they are becoming even more acute and responsive. Sensory indicators, from the eye or ear, journey first from the brain to the thalamus, and then to the amygdala. Another signal is then transported to the neocortex (the thinking part of the brain). The initial reaction enables the amygdala (emotive/reactive part of the brain) to react sooner than the thinking brain as the amygdala was implanted for survival purposes. The neocortex takes longer as it is more logical, rational and comprehends information until it is completely refined and tailored to fit our values and beliefs. Emotions are quicker to gather and more effective when an instantaneous and immediate response is necessary (especially when reacting in a fight or flight mode) whereas the neocortex comes to the forefront (no pun intended) when deep thought, detail and consideration are required. Emotions are pure sensations whereas thoughts require detail, specifics and formation.

In order to comprehend our emotions, we must explore the art of motivation. Motivation is the desire to take action. People are either motivated by fear (feeling that they may not be enough, or feeling like they may lose something), or by the prospect of greater gain (knowing they are enough, yet still wanting to acquire more). There is a massive difference between the two. For instance, the thought, "What will my future physical self be like?" can actually spark two reactions: you will either feel motivated by the fear of gaining more fat (fearful motivation), or you will become motivated by the potential of losing more fat (gainful motivation). Most people operate out of fear. The best financial investors (and physical investors) always protect the downside (damage control), but to be truly happy in life, we must experience more pleasure from really succeeding physically than the pain of potentially gaining more fat.

We cannot prevent all poor quality thinking, as it is simply part of being human. However, we can choose to remain indifferent to these thoughts. We will want to detach any emotion from our negative notions, and pump energy (emotion) into our more empowering ideas. So, for instance, if we think of something that cannot support us, then we must purposefully make the effort to shift our attention. We must not attach physical movement to these thoughts (hitting a desk, covering our faces, holding ourselves tightly, biting our nails etc.), as they can strengthen our emotional response to these negative thoughts, and thus engrain them more deeply within us. Become indifferent to these thoughts. For example, if the thought comes to your mind that you will never lose the weight that you want, then simply sit still indifferently, and instead appease this negativity by feeling grateful for your current shape; focus on the things that you can do to change your situation, and attach stronger physical movements to these empowering thoughts. You can then purposely choose to think, "I am enough as I am, and I can put myself in different situations to develop the kind of body I really want," and then you can add some form of intense physical movement (fist pump, nodding fervently, exhaling intensely etc.), so that this idea is more emotionally captivating.

If we ask questions with enough passion, enthusiasm and emotive language, then the answers will soon appear. Weakly phrased questions delivered tediously will induce frail, fragile responses whereas open, positively phrased

58

questions will cultivate potent, empowering solutions. There is a momentous difference between, "How will I make sure that I don't gain any more weight?" and "How can I significantly change my confidence, body, energy and life?" Think about the words you use, and whether you are focusing on what you want rather than what you do not want.

"Your beliefs become your thoughts, Your thoughts become your words, Your words become your actions, Your actions become your habits, Your habits become your values, Your values become your destiny." - Mahatma Gandhi

Setting up a successful pattern (thought, emotion, action) starts with the smallest of things. We can then work our way up. The smaller things we accomplish can sometimes foreshadow the larger things to come. Our thoughts trigger other thoughts; our emotions trigger other emotions; our behaviours trigger other behaviours. Many, if not all, of our actions are linked to one another. Everything within us flows from one thing to another. If we want to change a behaviour, then we must first analyse the surrounding behaviours that occur both beforehand and thereafter. If we want to stop eating unhealthy foods, then what actions usually take place leading up to the act of smoking? What happens after we eat unhealthily that makes it so strongly engrained in our action-based repertoire? For example, do we bite our nails (because we emotionally thought about something), and then at a cake, which was then followed by a more relaxed conversation over the phone? These physical actions are oftentimes sequentially habitual. They must all be evaluated and changed if we really want one to change in particular.

"We are what we repeatedly do. Excellence, then, is not an act, but a habit." - Aristotle

How can we begin to transform a negative habit into one that is more supportive? We must, firstly, be aware of something if we are to change a negative trio pattern. This is known as conscious incompetence. Catch yourself making the error. This initially breaks the pattern even if we continue to make the mistake in future. By just making it explicit to us, it sets the change in motion. Subsequently, we can literally act out this same negative pattern on purpose when a similar event occurs, as it will serve to emphasise the folly of its enactments. Once we play with the emotions associated with the actions, then we can take control of our feelings and detach from these actions. In addition, we can also practice improving our own reactions and patterns by changing how we react when another person makes an error. For example, if we get angry with ourselves when we accidentally smash a glass, then we can start to correct this harsh perception by changing your response when another person accidentally smashes a glass. It conditions us to react more favourably, so that we choose more uplifting ways of treating ourselves. This shift will improve our thoughts, emotions and behaviours in other areas also such as health and fitness.

Furthermore, internal representations are also important. Part of successfully changing a pattern, or our perceptions, is to detach ourselves from the actual experience. This enables us to comprehend how our brains usually work (automatic response) when in the moment. We begin to play with the relationship between our thoughts and emotions. For example, if we want to eat healthily, yet we are about to be offered a really 'tasty' yet unhealthy cake by our friends, then the following pattern might occur.

Thought: "Don't even think about it. I know it looks good. Looking at it isn't helping! I guess it will look bad if I am not having some with the others, and I can always burn it off later. Why can't I ever just say, no?"

Emotion: Disappointment.

Action: Eating the cake, which is then followed by tense, closed, sunken body language, lack of eye contact and so on.

A strong emotion is tied to this: fear. This fear then overwhelms the immediate experience; we become exceedingly focused on the inside (ourselves), and what we are thinking. Our internal dialogue shifts from being about an experience with our friends (external) to being totally focused on what we are doing. This sequence of events become so engrained that it is exactly the process that takes over when in the same or similar situations. However, we can interrupt this pattern: "Actually, so what if I don't eat unhealthily just because it's expected of me? If my friends cannot support me, then things are obviously not as good as they should be." Our new emotion might be one of peacefulness or self-acceptance. Our new actions may take the form of rejecting any future unhealthy offerings, showing relaxed and confident body language, and most importantly, staying focused on the present moment with our friend rather than immersed in our own little negative dialogue.

The sequencing of particular thoughts, emotions, and actions solidifies and intensifies every time it takes place. It has a domino effect. Positively, good things can occur, and positive language can be reinforced, which perpetuates our mental fortitude. We may say that we are successful at this or that. Then our beliefs in this aptitude transcends into an ability to learn and grow in another subject or discipline. The meta-belief then becomes, "I can succeed wherever I put my attention." Our paradigms shifts, and our belief systems alter. Small things accumulate and transform into larger structures. These larger structures, now programmed into our subconscious, determine our core beliefs. We begin to move toward and attract healthier actions and situations. Liking takes place in the conscious; love develops in the subconscious. Sadness takes place in the conscious; depression pervades the subconscious. A subconscious pattern is shaped through the repetition of conscious thoughts, feelings and actions. The cycle continues. Generally, our subconscious dictates our actions and behaviour.

Incredible things can happen when the subconscious works to help fulfil our goals. The conscious is at the water's surface; the subconscious lies deep in the sea. The conscious is the tree; the subconscious is the roots. If we water the roots, then the tree shall grow, but if we neglect the roots, the tree will wither and die or cease to grow at all. I am reminded of the Chinese Bamboo tree. This spectacular tree is wonderfully unique. If we were to water this tree's seeds, it would not even grow an inch within one year, nor would it grow at all the second or third... It is in the fourth year, of constant watering, that the tree begins to grow substantially and monumentally. Not only does this tree begin to grow, but within just a few short weeks it can grow up to ninety feet tall! Astonishing. Think of your life in this way. Our roots and seeds need constant care, support and attention. If we suddenly achieve something fantastic, trust me, more often than not, it happened because of changes we began to make a while ago. Once we have laid the foundations, marvelous and incredulous things can develop. We always need to get to the root of the problem!

Mind and Body

"To keep the body in good health is a duty... otherwise we shall not be able to keep our mind strong and clear." - Buddha

Emotions are the intermediaries between mind and body. Our mind thinks of something, our emotions are stimulated by these thoughts, and our body acts and reacts accordingly. The body, our form, is a physical expression of how our minds function. If we want to remain calm, and have fewer physical illnesses, then partake in yoga and meditation. If we want to be mentally open and flexible, then stretch frequently, and keep the body agile. If we want to be mentally strong and assertive, then lift heavier weights or train more intensely. The mind can dictate how the body operates, and the body can dictate how the mind operates. Sharpen both mind and body, so that they continue to support one another.

What are the differences between our thoughts and emotions? An emotion can be seen as an energetic thought that has not yet been mentally processed granularly and accurately enough to become a complete meticulous, distilled thought. The unknown (an emotion) is then the intermediary between a thought and an action. Uncertainty then becomes the driving force that powers us to go from a thought to taking action. Unlike an emotion, a thought is precise and definable. An action is a reaction to strong emotion. An action can be seen as trying to achieve a result of one kind or another. Perhaps actions want to make sense of something. Actions can therefore be seen as movements that derive from unspecific thoughts; it is the desire for clarity that we take action.

When people are highly sensitive and emotional, they lack clarity, and so often seek solidarity in a strong, authority figure (someone more certain, logical and more thoughtful). Interestingly, we experience more sensations per minute than thoughts. Perhaps this is because sensations and emotions are easier to feel than thoughts are to think. Why? Thoughts require accuracy, meticulousness and clarity whereas emotions require a plethora of information that has not been ruminated or granularly broken down. An emotion's indefinable nature keeps it intriguing and influential. If we want to become less emotional, then we must become more thoughtful.

Purely feeling and reacting takes away our control. Emotions are not in any sense futile or less valuable as they function to drive us to do things. This is why a healthy balance between thoughts and emotions are necessary. The purely emotional person physically does a lot, but does not get anywhere whereas the extreme thinker does not get anywhere either because all they do is just think. There is a time to think, and there is a time to feel. However, once we take the time to think an emotion through thoroughly, we take back control, and the emotion becomes thoughts. We now have control of our actions. This is why, in many ways, it can be beneficial to really break down the steps of any negative emotions we experience. This may not be as necessary for our positive emotions as we conspicuously want to sustain our energy in these areas!

People will either experience a form of negativity leading up to unhealthy eating or after having eaten something they feel guilty about. We must understand when we experience negativity and why. In order to change a negative emotion, we must be able to trace it back to its most fundamental origination. All negative thinking can be traced back to an element of fear. Let us consider revisit the example of being offered cake by our friends. These are some of the questions we would have wanted to ask ourselves. Why have I been offered cake? It is a way of building trust and rapport. Why does it build trust and rapport? Because it is a pleasant offering that is supposed to bring some form of pleasure. Why does it provide pleasure? Because it tastes good. Why does it taste good? Because it contains addictive and mostly artificial ingredients. Why does it contain these? So that we become addicted, and buy it more often. Why must we buy it more often? Because that is one way of how our lifestyles are controlled. Why must our lifestyles be controlled? Because its harder to be sold lots of things if we have emotional control. Why is that harder? Because our associations are controlled, which allows us to make better choices. Why should we make better choices? So that we can stay focused on our goals and not be led down less supportive avenues. We have broken down the emotions we experience in this situation into only thought processes, which takes away a lot of the emotional connection we might have with this experience. This will make us feel more in control of what we eat.

If we break negative emotions down like this, then we realise what we must do. We learn more about ourselves, and how we function, which provides greater control. We can easily identify when and why we experience negative emotions, and trace them down to our deep underlying beliefs. However, we must be totally honest with ourselves if this is to work powerfully. Emotions are only useful if they incentivise us to go for what we want in life. The person who knows why they feel the way they do has control of it, but pure thought, without emotion, will not allow us to use this feeling to drive an action.

An action is never random. An action is never separate. Even actions that we think are random and impulsive have emotions attached to them. A random action is a reaction to the desire for something different for instance. Thoughts, feelings, actions and circumstances continuously flow from one to the next. They go around and around, always changing, our moods ceaselessly shifting, building upon one another or changing completely due to a particular incident. Our emotion is the catalyst: it is the fuel that turns our thoughts into actions. The way we live our lives is a reflection of how the brain works. If bad things happen to us frequently, then dreadful things operate in our brains. If we often eat unhealthily, then stressful things operate in our minds, and stress is a form of fear. If we understand this, then we begin to look at unhealthy eating and being in bad shape as something rather disappointing and uninspiring. This is the mindset we need in order to have the fuel and energy to stay in great shape.

As the old saying goes, "Everything happens for a reason." Everything is synchronised as shared by the brilliant psychologist: Carl Jung. If we are accumulating success in several avenues of our lives, then it is a reflection of our successful thinking. The mind's clarity and purity will enable us to make the right decisions and, thus, remain impervious to any disease we were predisposed to possibly acquire. We must defend the mind from entropy and the detrimental patterns that subjugate hope and health.

What leads to the creation of metal impairment before it becomes a physical disease? Stress. Stress is the biggest culprit. What is stress? Stress is often what happens when we become excessively drawn into our lives, and we fail to step back in order to view our lives from afar. It is the detrimental disharmony and discord within us. Stress is what happens when we take on too much mentally or physically at a certain time. Stress occurs when we feel overwhelmed. Stress is a form of anxiety; stress therefore a form of fear. Fear is therefore our biggest enemy; it is the biggest killer in life. We must address the different types of fear we experience, and link these to how they affect our health and physical bodies.

The Ego

"You can either be a host to God, or a hostage to your ego." – Wayne Dyer

Our egos are massively tied to our habits and beliefs, which must be addressed if we are to rewire the way our brains work, so that we can change our health and bodies. We all get humbled in life. We all have an ego, and to be fair, to an extent, it is necessary to have an ego otherwise we will not be bothered about improving the quality of our lives. However, we must either check our own egos (know that even though we are fantastic, quality human beings, we are not that special in the grand scheme of things), or life will humble our egos for us (we might get into an accident; we might be cheated on; we might lose all our wealth etc.). Change the internal, and the external shall change. We must not want something too badly as it can make us choke (metaphorically at least). As Wayne Dyer elicits, we can want something, but we must not be attached to it. Enjoy the process leading up to success. Happiness is a journey; it is not a destination. If we only feel happy once we have accomplished something, then we will only experience true happiness for very short glimpses in our lives, if any at all.

We must be brutally honest with ourselves. Some people cannot be true to themselves usually because their ego is in the way. The ego can sometimes protect us. However, it is far more perilous if we fail to dig deep enough to uncover the latent and pervasive thoughts that truly exist. Every time we get angry, it is our egos controlling us. This requires us to understand that we are imperfect, and we must know that we will never be perfect. Having the attitude that we are continuous learners who will never be complete will ensure that we maintain high standards and that we are ever improving. Happiness can be defined as feeling and knowing that we are progressing in something that is a priority to us. This priority can be anything: being gregarious, creative, giving, affluent, intellectual, and so forth. If it is important to us, then we must be developing that side of our lives in order to thrive.

Everything that has happened to us thus far has been the right thing to happen for on our particular journeys. Though this may not be apparent and conspicuous now, or ever for that matter, we should know that everything has happened to make us who we are today. Choose love rather than fear. When we experience love in the present moment, then we cannot be fearful, stressed or anxious because love is the most impregnable and impervious experience that it overwhelms all other insufficiencies. Love is therefore the main way to overcome the ego. It is the best way to alleviate the pressure that results in unhealthy eating and living.

A balance must be made between giving energy to our egos (feeling unique, special and significant) and our superego (being humble, virtuous, respectful, giving).

Once we go one way or the other between these two conceivably distinct stratums, then we either become too serene and passive or overtly narcissistic, greedy and cynical. The ability to float between these intrinsic perspectives enables abundance, awareness and excellence. Obviously, there are times in life when we will need to market and sell ourselves (the ego): when getting a job, attracting investors, persuading our children, attracting a partner etc. However, we also need to understand that our lives in this world will soon be over, and we are practically nothing in the context of this world and nature. Approach everything with an open and growth mindset. It is important to truly believe that we can accomplish anything in life. All it takes is great discipline, energy, a drive to continuously learn, and a healthy attitude to supposed 'failure.' The moment we say something cannot be attained, then we are correct. We limit our experiences and aptitudes by initially stating that we are not good at something or that we could never be good at it. We must know that we can change our health and bodies drastically if we have the right mindset, and if we take consistent action to support our health goals.

Our egos are responsible for being judgemental and for stereotyping. When we label or judge someone or something, we limit the potential to notice other things about them. We will literally look for things that support our initial judgements, and our ability to perceive alternatively will be blocked. There is nothing wrong with stereotyping instantly (because this is a way to condense knowledge or perceived knowledge quite rapidly). However, it is very important to be open minded, and to be willing to change your assumptions if presented with new information. In many ways, this relates to the ego, as people do not like to see many talents within the same person as it makes them feel inadequate. We must break the limiting belief that tells us that we must compromise something (such as our health and body) if we are to have a successful career or family for example. This is wrong, as we can be successful in all key areas in life.

The ego is necessary in that it is our driving force as it relates to the 'survival of the fittest.' It is the part within us that thinks we are special, unique and powerful. It is a necessary component of life, but must be kept in check like all things. We must feel as though we are special whilst also believing that every other person is just as worthy in his or her own way. Everyone has a gift to give the world. Every person has different priorities, relationships, coping mechanisms, interests, experiences and so forth. How could we possibly expect or look down upon someone for being different? Unfortunately, the ego can backfire on us. Our egos trick us into believing that we are greater than we really are, and we all, in our own ways, are humbled one way or another. The ego breaks on many occasions. The more egotistical and materialistic we are, the higher our ego shall climb, and so the fall shall be far more devastating and immobilising. Everything will work out for us in life if we simply get out of the way. Having to always be right immediately makes us wrong.

The stronger our egos are, the harder it is to self-reflect.

Perhaps the ego was a biological creation in order to keep us alive: a survival instinct and adaptation. The obsession with the ego (feeling superior, feeling significant and feeling unique) is what keeps us moving forward and immersed in our own experience, which is both worthy and wicked. The ego can therefore be seen as the ultimate creation due to our fear of death. Death and ego are always in conflict. In order to be self-reflective, we must therefore detach ourselves from the ego, and this is unnatural, as the ego was created to combat death. If we are changing our personality (which we all must do by changing our thoughts, emotions and behaviours – the entire point of reading this book), then we will inevitably face resistance by our ego as it associates change (the unknown) with death: our ultimate fear. However, for us to really learn and change our current situation, we must be able to self-reflect, and so we must be able to detach ourselves from our egos. Let us therefore analyse how our egos hurt us, so that we can reduce its influence on us to some degree, thereby, enabling us to self-reflect, and make the necessary changes to improve our bodies and health.

Fear and the Ego

"The ego is the false self-born out of fear and defensiveness." - John O'Donohue

Let us consider the many ways in which we hold ourselves back, and begin to analyse our own decisions, actions and current situations. One of the main struggles people have is their inability to realistically reflect on their current strengths and areas for improvement. What is it that holds us back? Fear. Fear holds us back. Fear can save your life. Unfortunately, fear can also create a life unworthy of being saved.

People lie to themselves as a way of protecting their egos. They might make themselves appear as though they do not need anything, when in reality it is the thing they need most. Here is a fitting analogy around fitness: the exercise you least enjoy doing at the gym is the one your mind and body need to do most. So why do people find it hard to be honest with themselves about their circumstance? They are simply too immersed in their own lives. Like a rat in the rat race, they are too narrow-minded and fixated on purely what they see in front of them. They never take the time to step back and view the consequences of their limiting thoughts, negative feelings and ineffective actions. They convince themselves that things happen to them, and it is not their fault. They convince themselves that they do not need to improve, and that improving is for the weak and vulnerable. They have brainwashed themselves into believing that their way is the right and only way.

Conversely, these blinded individuals may just be extremely apathetic. Change and reflection requires objectivity, energy and focus. It is easy to look at others and focus on their faults, but when people do this, it is often a form of procrastination, as they do not wish to work on themselves. Unfortunately, self-reflection requires a humble, honest approach. It requires the ability to think, "I am not amazing at this or that, and I want to improve, so I will be seeking help from others one way or another." The following example of inner dialogue are negatively phrased to truly illustrate how a person's mind might work, and how habits can be changed through persistent questioning:

"Why don't you exercise more?"
"Because I do not value being pretentious and focusing on looking good."
"Why don't you value looking good?"
"Because I value the mind more."
"Why do you value the mind more?"
"Because the mind is the most important thing."
"Why is the mind the most important thing?"
"Because it does all your thinking and determines your future."
"How does it determine your future?"
"Because you can think things through and plan things out."
"Why do you want to plan things out?"
"Because I don't want to make mistakes."
"Why don't you want to make mistakes?"
"Because I don't want negative things in my life, and I don't want people to judge me because of my mistakes."
"Why don't you want negative things in your life?"
"Because I wouldn't know how to react."
"Why wouldn't you know how to react?"
"Because I'm not that mentally flexible and positive."
"How can you be more flexible and positive?"
"By reducing stress, and being able to relax."
"How can you reduce stress and be more relaxed?"
"By exercising more."

This example foregrounds the importance of questioning everything we do. The honest answer to the above dilemma is as follows: "I'm lazy when it comes to exercise

74

because, deep down, I know I will never be able to compete with others in this field, so I reject its importance. It's easier for me to stay as I am, and refute the truth even though it would make me a better, happier person. I guess it's just my ego getting in the way, preventing me from progressing." The things we find the hardest to do are the things we need to do the most. The ability to think and self-reflect is of monumental significance. Our ego, left unattended, is our biggest enemy. We all have, or have had, false paradigms and perceptions that veneer the truth. Self-reflecting, and being brutally honest with ourselves, will prevent us from experiencing copious affliction again and again. We all have challenging things happen to us, and we possibly felt that they were undeserved. We felt we could not make sense of why it had to happen to us. If we still cannot conjure a positive spin on why a bad thing occurred, then we must at least understand that there is a message currently indiscernible to us. We must be careful with what we expose our eyes and ears to, as it dictates our focus, and therefore our thoughts. We find what we seek. We can use any challenge as a way of strengthening our resolve as it relates to our health and bodies.

"I'm not afraid of dying. I'm afraid not to have lived." - Wim Hof

In order to have the life we want, we must stretch ourselves and conquer these dragons (more often than not they are not fierce dragons, but puppies masquerading as dragons). If people fear many things (they experience stress, anxiety, worry and are quite rigid), then they must learn to love and give more to themselves and others:

when we love, we cannot fear. Why fear when we can love? When we experience love in the present moment, then it is impossible to fear anything. Therefore, love as much and as often as we can. Love our families; appreciate our friends; give to charities; share our skills with strangers. Our existence on earth in this form is limited, so we must go for what we want. Dream big and live abundantly. It is never too late to change and thrive. This is why we must set exceedingly high standards around our health and physical goals. We never know what we are capable of until we push the boundaries.

Stress

"It's not stress that kills us, it is our reaction to it." - Hans Selye

Stress is probably the biggest thing that ruins most people's health and fat-loss goals. What is stress? It is intangible. Stress is an internal representation. To experience stress is to create disharmony within. Therefore, we create stress. We choose to experience stress based on the things we think we should do or what we might have to do. Stress is pressure. It is a build-up of all the things that we supposedly need to get done that do not appear pleasurable. So why do we choose to experience stress, and to release such toxic and radical reactions in our minds and bodies? Stress can be seen as responsible for all illnesses and diseases. It is the ultimate killer of lives. We must be able to notice when we are stressed on a daily or weekly basis, and have routines in place to best reduce this stress. Consider the things you do to reduce stress, and whether this actually creates stress in other ways. Do your utmost to utilise positive, supporting stress-reducing activities to support your health, joy and self-esteem.

Is stress at all good for us? Hormesis is when we have to deal with a little bit of stress as a way of strengthening our will. Exercise is a form of hormesis. Therefore, we can never totally eliminate stress, but only engaging in minor stress will be beneficial. If stress levels rise too high, then that is when less desirable effects arise. When we truly experience nature we cannot be stressed. Living in an urban, busy city can make it harder, but we must enjoy nature where possible. Seeing, hearing and smelling the sea, trees, grass and so on can really put things into perspective. I am aware that this is a very romantic ideal, but enjoying the most basic, natural things in life will always alleviate stress.

We all struggle with stress to varying degrees. Everyone in life has their own coping mechanisms: exercising, driving, talking, socialising, arguing, sex, over-eating, under-eating, emotional eating, OCD and so forth. Choose more productive methods of releasing stress. Many people choose to self-harm: smoking, alcohol, illicit, or even licit, drugs and so on. Positive stress relievers are far more beneficial: exercise, martial arts training, sex, meditation and yoga. These experiences can increase the state of flow whilst simultaneously keeping mind and body robust. Even things like conversations, going for walks etc. are better choices. It is a choice that we all have, and one we are all accountable. Even though we all encounter moments of stress, we must embed positive stress-mitigating practices that will serve to relieve stress. We must enhance the general quality of our lives, by doing what we enjoy, such as playing golf or tennis, which do not have any repercussions, and which do not exacerbate stress, depression and illness.

We must take care of ourselves first. Only when we are happy are we truly in the right position to give to others freely and openly. We can only successfully take care of others in the long term, if we take care of ourselves first. Admittedly, we may be able to do nice things for others even if we are unhappy. However, we will become resentful or worse, and we will end up taking our frustrations out on people even closer to us, or people who will put up with our tempers. Some people sacrifice their own enjoyment in order to give to someone else. This altruistically loving, yet potentially self-righteous behaviour, will manifest itself in some other form of conflict and negative act in the future unless we are happy and content with ourselves. If we have short-tempers, then we should reflect upon this cycle of stress and whether we, in a way, add stress (anxiety and pressure) on top of stress in a kind of self-destructive cycle. What do we think about before we lash out? How can we better control our emotions? Our habits create our character. Do our habits induce affliction for others and ourselves, or do they inspire, motivate and catapult us, and others, to another level?

Ideally, we want to release stress in the healthiest ways. There is no need to take our stress out on others in the form of passive aggression or arguing or starting a fight or looking for someone to make a mistake, so that we can embarrass him or her. Others will appreciate our emotional intelligence if we remove our stress more appropriately. Firstly, we must consider what happens when we get stressed. What can we do to reduce stress? Can we be more proactive and plan better? Can we train our minds to expect stress on certain days or in certain situations? Can we seek support from others to reduce stress? Secondly, consider the ways in which we release stress, and assess how this empowers or disempowers us. Stress is not necessarily a bad thing. However, too much stress can be overwhelming, and it makes us lose all sense of control. Therefore, it might prove useful to evaluate what we could control, and what things will work out just fine if we are unable to control them. After all, stress is a loss of control. The more controlling we are, the more inclined we are to experience high levels of stress: we are dealing with others in life who also want a sense of control. We are not responsible for other people's actions. As long as we can control our own, then we should feel a great deal of pride and pleasure from determining our health and physical appearances.

"The greatest weapon against stress is our ability to choose one thought over another." – William James

Mistakes

"You build on failure. You use it as a stepping stone. Close the door on the past. You don't try to forget the mistakes, but you don't dwell on it. You don't let it have any of your energy, or any of your time, or any of your space." - Johnny Cash

Unhelpfully reacting to our mistakes will also add to our debilitating mindset, which indirectly ruins our health and body. Making mistakes can also detrimentally affect our emotions, and our emotions are always responsible for what and how we eat. Mistakes often happen when overwhelmed (stressed), psychologically beaten or when the mind becomes sloppy. Our mistakes should reveal the need to bring order to the mind's chaos in order to provide the clarity needed to perform at one's best. Moreover, mistakes derive from ineffectively dealing with our problems. People tend to be more forgetful when there is a lack of mental clarity. It is fundamental to understand what mistakes show us, and where our attention must go if we are to eradicate any future unnecessary struggles that can negatively affect our health and how we hold onto existing fat. Interestingly, once we make a mistake, it is easier to make mistakes either within that same field or within another. Why? Uncertainty and self-doubt pervade the subconscious. Because we are being harsh on ourselves for making mistakes, we then trip ourselves up more often as pondering over the mistake attracts additional errors. Once we allow something to own our thoughts and feelings, it becomes easier to be owned in other areas. This rippling and crippling effect occurs because of negative perceptions.

Mistakes often occur as a result of being lopsided. When we always follow our strengths and avoid our weaknesses, we become more inflexible in our approach to things. We become susceptible and weaker because our foundations are not robust enough. There is a time to be assertive and aggressive; there is a time to be spontaneous and outgoing; there is a time to sit in silence and ponder; there is a time to show love and affection; there is a time for experiencing pain. One of our greatest assets can easily become a major weakness; our greatest weakness may in fact become our biggest strength. Sometimes the greatest thing to ever happen to us is the thing that brings us the greatest pain. We must not immerse ourselves in its experience, but learn the lessons that are always there. Contemplate how and why it brought us pain. Our pain shows where our energy must go (but not stay in!).

We are constantly changing physically, never to be the same again. However, we often struggle to accept change mentally. Yes, a certain level of mental change is inevitable in a world where experiences and situations are never exactly replicable, and so slight adjustments can be made. The body changes drastically from childhood to adulthood to an elderly age, but one thing remains: most people are still afraid to change their perceptions, paradigms and belief systems due to fear. However, it is the act of pushing through our comfort level that fulfils our deep desire for progression. People usually create negative experiences and emotions in order to stay where they are. They choose to experience anger, sadness or guilt to ensure that they do not have to do more fundamental work that is necessary to progress as a person. They think, "I'm angry right now," so the last thing they want to do is exercise, or eat a salad or reflect upon their current goals. Ignorance and stubbornness can keep us stagnant and thus depressed. Our mistakes demonstrate the need for greater flexibility. If we are making mistakes in any avenue, then we must become more flexible.

Every situation can be interpreted positively, even though it appears negative or destructive at the surface level. Getting fired from a job could be the event that provides the impetus to start that long-awaited business that could free you and thus indirectly positively affect your fat-loss. Infidelity taught you that you needed a better quality partner, or to escape when you did as it perhaps saved you a lifetime of limitations and conflict. Seek to find the positive in everything that happens. It allows us to take on more, and thus grow more. If small problems are perceived as big problems, then we will never have the wherewithal to attack the bigger things in life. The more stress we can handle or mitigate, the more we can take on and thus accomplish. Our inner energy, that which is intangible, dictates our circumstance and happenings. There are energy sources indiscernible to us. The mistakes we make were supposed to happen. They are small signs for us to change what we are doing. The real pain is not in the mistakes we make, but in our inability to learn from these mistakes.

We learn a lot about people's characters by how they deal with smaller things. How a person resolves their problems reflects how they conduct their lives, how they filter things mentally, and present things to themselves mentally to mitigate the damage. Unfortunately, it is all too easy for people to fail in life, and point the finger. The harder thing is to develop the resilience needed to stay in the fight, and refusing to lose until we eventually win. The same applies to our physical shape. There will be times where you feel like you deserve better physical results, but we must keep going and subtly tweak things along the way. We will get there, but we must enjoy the process.

"It is not over until I win." – Les Brown

Refuse to stop because of consternation. Depression develops as a result of learned helplessness, and labelling oneself as a victim. Unfortunately, many people choose to be the victim because it is the easy way out. We must take responsibility for our circumstances. People are ignorant because they choose to be. People are ignorant because they are afraid of the truth; they are afraid of the other. Our ignorance allows us to keep making mistakes. Ignorance is oftentimes the ego at play. In order to progress, we must distance ourselves from the familiar. Familiarity is a trap, even if it is a good habit. Whatever omniscient power exists, know that it is interminably testing us. We cannot control every single experience in our lives, but we can always control how we perceive things. Our perceptions are vital for establishing how we view ourselves, and what our standards are.

We must spot our mistakes earlier rather than later to avoid any significant damage physically or emotionally. We can spot the simple signs of faltering attention or ineffectual thinking by even the most minutia of instances. Again, it may seem like over-thinking and hyperbole, but small things always creep up on us until something major happens. Maybe getting injured at the gym highlighted just how busy and overly mentally occupied we could have been. These smaller scale issues and irrational actions illustrate the need for either something to be enhanced or something to be lessened. Take the time to reflect, learn and come back with greater fortitude.

Very early in life we develop powerful belief systems often involuntarily based on what we saw all around us especially through the actions of those who raised us. "Jake, don't run!" "Jake be careful because you know what will happen." "Jake you cannot do that." "Be careful" or "Don't drop that!" or "This is serious, so do it right." Inadvertently, the parent is setting their child up for uncertainty and limitations. Be vigilant, yet assertive. Be calculated, yet practical. Our risk-taking ability and confidence can become diminished over time because of what we choose to hear and accept as truth. We must question our deepest paradigms and indoctrinations, but that does not necessarily mean we must always change them. Simply become inquisitive. We must question our beliefs around our health, and the story we tell ourselves about what our bodies should look like and why.

How we react to our mistakes and failures determine the amount of mental and emotional success we will have with our fat loss goals in the long term. The person who was dieting for several weeks and lost no weight for some reason can do one of a few things: break down, admit defeat and vow to never attempt to eat healthily again, which builds an entire web of fear, a bubble that limits growth, or they can utilise different strategies and seek advice from others. Maybe you were distracted, less prepared or took the process too seriously, and you got in your own way by thinking too much. You learn most about someone when they supposedly fail than when he or she wins. We should not be evaluated by our successes, but by our reactions to perceived failures. It is in adversity where we are truly challenged, not when we win or achieve the goal. Effectively responding to our mistakes, and reducing how many times we make the same mistakes, will directly affect how we feel, and thus how we show up in terms of our eating and training.

Procrastination

"Only put off until tomorrow what you are willing to die having left undone." – Pablo Picasso

People often procrastinate when things seem challenging. Why not just start the healthy eating tomorrow as the party is tonight? Why go to the gym when we can fix that cabinet in the house that has needed to fixed for a long time now? Why have that cold shower in the morning that develops your discipline for the entire day when you can just leave for work a little earlier? Distractions impede our concentration and clarity. Procrastination, problems, and mistakes are all related. Some people procrastinate by opting to choose negative feelings; they make excuses as to why they never make it to the next step: "I feel bad, so I do not have to work harder." "I feel awful right now, so I don't need to exercise." "I feel lethargic right now, so why should I bother having that cold shower?" These are often excuses made to protect the ego. No one wants to admit that they cannot achieve, thereby hurting one's ego, and so they manifest negative feelings, which almost always include external factors. They excuse themselves from not having to improve, and it prevents them from doing what they should do: training harder at the gym; consistently eating healthy meals; embedding quality routines that increase our metabolism and so on. Some find excuses to do things or not do things: "I have a meeting today that I am not looking forward to, so I am entitled to eat poorly and unhealthily." "My wife does not treat me the way she used to, so I need my comfort food for self love." If we look for excuses and reasons, then we will find them. These forms of justification have the same purpose in that they stop us from taking responsibility for our actions, and thus empower our weaknesses.

Having the ability to eat and exercise the way we want to do is incredible. However, firstly, we must become aware of how we procrastinate. Secondly, we must be able to overpower these detrimental habits by taking pressure off ourselves. If we know we need to eat healthily for the entire day, then we will do anything and everything to sabotage the process. If we know we have a daunting gym session that requires us to be at our best, then we will come up with excuses to do other things. This is why we must alleviate the pressure by saying, "I am just going to enjoy the process, and do what I can." Interestingly, we will consistently end up doing so much better simply because we lessened the pressure, which enabled our creativity to flourish whilst also increasing our energy levels. We will have an extra spring in our steps. We will want to give more. Why? Because we are defeating what is meant to be defeated. We take one step closer to achieving our mental and physical purpose. Starting the work every day is the hardest part. Getting up to train, have a cold shower and eat a healthy first meal sets the example for the entire day. If we show up consistently, then things will begin to work for us, and not just in the world of health. However, we always need to know *why* we want to accomplish these things. Ensure that your why is bigger than your own needs. For example, are you doing it for your family, so that they do not have to grow up with self-esteem issues later in life? Are you doing it so that you can end the depression and suffering that can stem from obesity and low energy for many helpless people?

We must know that we are always being tested. Once we take action and stop procrastinating, we will set a chain of events in motion. If we continue to grind daily, we will defeat procrastination, and develop the resolve needed to accelerate the quality of our health and body. Perhaps we all exert the same amount of energy: some use it to win; others use it to fail. Trouncing procrastination, and avoiding drama, will assist in bringing our dreams and desires into fruition. How do you procrastinate? Procrastination takes many forms. We may be conscious of some while others are insidiously running our lives. Why did we have that argument yesterday when we knew we had a deadline on Monday that required our absolute attention? OCD in itself can actually be a form of procrastination: why do we inundate the mind with incessant and compulsive cleaning when we have far more demanding and worthwhile endeavours to pursue? It does not matter how or where we were bitten, what matters is that we were poisoned.

Our Emotional Home

"That's the thing about depression: A human being can survive almost anything, as long as she sees the end in sight. But depression is so insidious, and it compounds daily, that it's impossible to ever see the end." - Elizabeth Wurtzel

We all have an emotional home. It is the preponderant emotion we experience. Our emotional home refers to the main governing emotion that we experience most often. We can improve our relationships with others, as well as ourselves, if we understand the core emotion people choose to experience: some people tend to get angry in order to take action; some people do everything they can to be relaxed; some people tend to worry more than anything else in order to keep active. This is the main emotion we tend to experience when on autopilot. Whenever we are not consciously thinking, this is where our subconscious leads us. It is our 'default modes.' If we know our emotional home, then we can understand how this affects the way we eat and exercise. We can access this state in order to motivate us, as they are the emotions we have learned to feel in order to get things done. The problem is people often do not access this state when it comes to health endeavours, which creates a disconnection: they do not feel gravitated to these healthy activities because they are not putting themselves in their traditional state. For example, if our emotional home is one of anger, and when you become angry, you eat unhealthily, then we must condition ourselves to eat healthy foods when we are angry. People who feel angry have conditioned themselves to eat unhealthy foods rather than better alternatives. We must either change our emotional home or change what we do when we access this state.

Experiencing a positive or negative emotion frequently enough will inevitably lead to a longer-term emotional state. Depression derives from experiencing moments of sadness so often that it takes its subconscious place as being the default experience. This is how a person can be around or with so many people, yet feel miserable and lonely inside. They might fleetingly experience a positive emotion, but their predominant emotion, dictated by their subconscious, is one of hopelessness. Depression exists when a person's present moments are impossible to be fully lived with joy and pleasure. If we are depressed, then even when we are doing something deemed enjoyable, we simply cannot because depression is the long-term, embedded emotion.

Happiness is of course the opposite, and it is also an overruling state. Any activity that comes our way can be approached positively. We can be washing the dishes, in a hostile environment, having had an altercation with someone, yet recognise that this moment will only bring discomfort or pain for a very short moment if at all! Happiness stems from experiencing joy and laughter recurrently meaning that it takes its subconscious role as being our default experience. This is how people often focus on good things when something seemingly upsetting has happened. The good news is we can program our minds until it falls into a certain automatic response. We want to love how we think, imagine and perceive things. While it may not appear so, we choose how we think and feel about any matter. We choose the grand state we wish to dominate our daily lives. Our habits and rituals determine the quality of our lives. Overcoming depression, and the ailments that come with it, cannot simply be achieved by taking part in fun and joyous activities alone. Instead of adding things, we may need to deduct other things. We can relinquish ourselves from the webs that entangle us, and from the depression that pervades our unconscious, and that negatively affects our fat-loss endeavours.

Fortunately, we can change our emotional centre by conditioning ourselves. Firstly, we must become aware of our emotional home. What emotions do you experience daily? We must be completely honest with ourselves if we are to make a profound difference. See if you can group certain emotions together if they are similar. Anxiety and worry are very similar. Joy and excitement are quite similar. Anger and frustration are quite similar. I am not talking about the way you portray yourself to strangers or the public because these are often inaccurate depictions of how we really feel. The way you interact with your friends, family and yourself are much more accurate. We can work toward embedding a positive preponderant emotion subconsciously by being honest with ourselves, and by admitting what it is that depresses us. This is how we take control of our issues and underlying pain. If we cannot pinpoint why we feel a certain way, then we cannot resolve the issue. This takes being incredibly honest with ourselves, which many people either cannot or do not want to do because it messes with our 'story.' Secondly, we must let go of the immobilising, reigning and overriding emotion that pervasively hinders the quality of our lives. We must forgive ourselves, and any others involved in what has deeply hurt us. We must learn to love ourselves, and feel empowered enough to transcend this debilitating feeling.

Secondly, it is beneficial to understand where this core emotion originated. What pain or pleasure may have influenced us to create this predominant emotion? Did something traumatic happen in your childhood? Is it the way a relationship ended? Is it from the teachings of a mentor? Is it what we experienced at school? Once we know the main things that shaped this core emotion, we can then make peace with these events. We can choose to let these past moments, or thoughts of the future, pass us, by changing what these events mean to us.

Thirdly, we can explicitly choose which core emotion we want to experience daily and often. We can then condition our past experiences, or perceptions of the future to match this new emotion. For example, if we are angry because a family member or friend betrayed us, then we can choose to forgive (internally) because we wish to live a peaceful life. If we do not trust people, because a previous business partner stole money from us, then we can be happy that this malevolent person is no longer part of our lives as he or she could have done even worse.

If we are always worrying about what is going to happen to us or people close to us, then we can choose to be grateful for all the things we or they have. Our past experiences and thoughts of the future have shaped our core emotion, yet we have the personal power to reframe these experiences and develop an uplifting portrayal of the future, so that we can experience more beautiful emotions frequently. We must overcome these emotional barriers if we are to make better, healthier choices for our minds and bodies.

Positivity is the water that can extinguish the fire. Love trumps hatred or anger every single time. Gratefulness suppresses fear every single time. Appreciation stifles anxiety every single time. Love yourself. Love others. Our biggest challenge is subduing the challenges within ourselves. Once we learn to control our inner demons, then we can focus on supporting others. We must be flexible in our thought; we must resist rigidity in our beliefs and abilities. Be open to new experiences and ways of perceiving events.

Perhaps every person is a good person, but because we do not understand how the mind works, we think that our biological, devilish thoughts are really who we are, and so people unfortunately act upon these. We may just get confused with what thoughts are ours, and what thoughts we should, or should not, empower. The only difference between a good and bad person is the thoughts they choose to follow. The more we decipher the thoughts that are biologically installed (more primitive and negative), then the more we can readily notice them and cast them aside. We then have the power to give light to our positive true selves. We have millions of thoughts every single day, and yet we only attach emotion to a certain amount. The more emotion we give to a thought, the more we are likely to take action in that specific direction. We must condition ourselves to dismiss our unsupportive thoughts, and champion the thoughts that we know to be our true selves. The better we understand how the mind works, the easier it will be to laugh at our negativity, and rightly choose more empowering thoughts that will support our health and body shape.

Whatever we believe becomes our truth. We are right no matter what we think because these are our overruling beliefs that dictate our journeys. Whatever we believe, we move toward. Whatever we move toward, we manifest in the physical form. Our natural gifts can be our biggest failures if left unconditioned. If we simply rely on our natural, inherent gifts, which we all have, then we can achieve life's purpose: striving to get better, to give more and to design our journeys most meaningfully. The beauty is in the process not in the accomplishment. Building your character is what brings true happiness. The results are what our egos gravitate toward, but it is not about that. It is about who we become. It is about how far we have travelled both literally and metaphorically. This is what we must learn to love about getting in the best shape of our lives: we must love the continual discipline, focus and energy we generate.

Let us consider how some people seem to know that they are in bad physical shape, and comprehend why they cannot change it. Why do some people enjoy their own pain or that of others for instance? Let us look at the brilliant ideas regarding meta-states as taught by Michael

Hall. There are often many emotions that are linked together, which makes it so much harder to decipher and change. The entire process becomes harder to entangle. One emotion is linked to a bigger emotion, which is then wrapped again in an even bigger emotion. Think of it as passing the baton in a relay race. For example, a person might experience fear or revulsion when they look at his or her body, which then triggers the need to rebel and do something outrageous. They rebel when they see or do the things that they fear. The feeling of rebellion is then wrapped within a larger emotion: excitement. They become excited when they rebel due to initially experiencing fear. A perilous pattern has been constructed. This pattern becomes engrained within his or her 'emotional system.' They then search for the familiar, and so seek opportunities that trigger this sequential emotional response and connection.

Let us consider another example. Have you ever felt embarrassed by something you said, or by the way in which you reacted to something? The feeling of embarrassment may become entangled with another emotion: anger. So you become angry because you felt embarrassed. This feeling of indignation can then get wrapped in another emotion: sadness. You may then become sad because of the anger you felt from being embarrassed. And there you have it. You have created a deeply embedded emotional pattern. We cannot simply look to change one emotion. We must understand the pattern we have created, and rewire it. We must break the emotions down, and change them one by one if the entire trio is to collapse. Ideally, it is better to start by changing the very first emotion we tend to experience.

We must supplant one emotion with another. We must choose a counteractive emotion that can succumb and encapsulate the preceding emotions in order to break this sequence of emotion (energy transference). We can break this pattern by disrupting it when we notice one of the emotions coming on. This can take the form of doing something outrageous as a way of stifling the emotional triggers. It can be helpful to become interested, fascinated or by simply being able to laugh at this unhelpful emotional response. For example, whenever you become embarrassed, then angry, and then sad, become fascinated by your sadness, or laugh at how you have become angry at such a silly incident that is meaningless in the grand scheme of things. When we can change our emotions, we can then act based on positive emotions or purely thoughts, which will enable us to make better choices as it relates to our health.

Everything in our internal and external world is analogous with water: they flow together seamlessly and ceaselessly. Everything in our lives is connected. Our thoughts are connected to our emotions, and our emotions are connected to our actions. Our actions trigger other sequences. Our subconscious is our long-term memory, which has unlimited storage and capacity whereas our conscious mind can only process between 3-7 different pieces of information. When we see life's fluidity (within our interactions with others and nature itself), then we can appreciate the beauty in its complexity. We do not have to tell ourselves that we must breathe in order to stay alive. It happens naturally. However, we can choose *how* we want to breathe to create different states. The brain works similarly. Our thoughts, feelings and actions work congruently, but you can decide *how*. Accept your thoughts; channel your emotions; act on your purpose.

People's Opinions

"Do not go where the path may lead, go instead where there is no path and leave a trail." - Carl Jung

We can listen to other people's opinions, but we can choose whether or not to accept what they say. Most people listen when someone gives them compliments, and when people notice what they are good at. The issue is that if we listen to people when they say good things about us, then we will also listen to people when they say bad things about us. I listen to everyone's opinions because I feel that we can learn something valuable from anyone. However, I choose to only accept the ideas of a few individuals and on certain matters where they are more proficient and experienced. Purposely, we should choose to not attach any emotion to what people say about us whether they are positive or negative because it is a form of indirect, and usually unintentional, manipulation. This is primarily because it is important to keep tabs on our egos whilst detaching ourselves from people's beliefs. Instead, write out your goals, remain focused on your path, and avoid what others say about what you are doing. We are not what others think of us; we are what we think of ourselves.

It takes courage to do what no one else around us is doing. It takes total certainty and belief in ourselves to step away from what the others do. If we listened to what others say, then we will be the same as everybody else: most people live unhealthily and without exceptional physiques. Why would you want to do the same as them? It takes great self-esteem to create your own path. This is true independence. People want to fit in so much that they actually jeopardise great mental and physical success in order to be the same, or similar, as those around them. We must set higher standards for ourselves, and hopefully those around us will follow their dreams, or simply we must simply allow others to continue on their own path. Never try to change someone. Simply model and allow.

Having the mentality that we must put ourselves first may appear egocentric and conceited, but it is the least selfish thing we can do. By making our bodies a priority, we develop the positive energy to want to make others feel good. Interestingly, living healthily is actually very altruistic because we tend to give more luxurious foods and treats to the other people with us. We do not want to share the pizza that was ordered for everyone. We want everyone else to enjoy it because we know that the pizza will not support our goals. Healthy individuals are not always looking to get a piece of what everyone is enjoying: we say no when biscuits are offered; we let everyone else enjoy the cakes or drinks given for free at the end of our meal at a restaurant. This is psychologically very helpful for us not just for our health, but for conditioning ourselves to believe that we have enough.

In order to live a healthy lifestyle, we must have an abundance mentality. If we think that the box of cookies is the last one on the planet, then we will want to scoff it down. Who cares if someone bought the most delicious desert for us? We can go and buy that desert any time we want. Why do you have to give in now? Scarcity thinking often results in poverty and ironically obesity. The two are linked in many ways. If we think that there are more than enough of the things we want in life (money, food, luxuries etc.), then we will not feel compelled to keep, eat and hoard things every chance we get.

Judgement

"The ability to observe without evaluating is the highest form of intelligence." - Jiddu Krishnamurti

In this section, we will be conditioning ourselves to release, or gradually release, the fear of being judged. The more drama we encourage in our lives, the more we become fixated with judging others and therefore being, or feeling, judged ourselves in other interactions. We must remove the urge to judge others, and thus become indifferent to the possible judgements others will make of us. The more we put ourselves out there, the more we will be judged. It is natural, and it is a good thing. You will never make everyone happy. Not wanting to be judged, results in not putting ourselves out of our comfort zones. Judgement goes back to being consumed by our reputation, and our reputation is linked to our ego. There is nothing wrong with projecting ourselves favourably, but the problem exacerbates exponentially when we stop taking action because we fear how we will be perceived. The more we suppress our desires and purpose, the more petulant, aggravated and depressed we become. We learn to put other people's opinions of ourselves above how we think and feel about ourselves. People with high self-esteem primarily care about what they think of themselves; people with low self-esteem are fixated on what others will think and feel about them. In order to fix these issues, we must start by changing our thoughts and emotions during smaller issues. If we care too much about how others perceive us when we are food shopping for instance, then these emotions proliferate and are strengthened when doing something more challenging such as approaching someone we really like or releasing artwork into the public domain. When we begin to change our focus when little things take place, we can indoctrinate ourselves helpfully and correct past conditioning. These notions will eventually seep into how we handle situations where the stakes are higher. We will have laid the foundations in our subconscious minds because of the many small incidents that we have worked on.

Constantly feeling as though we are being observed, scrutinised and judged makes many people remain inert. As children, we neither noticed nor cared about what strangers or our peers thought about us. We did what we wanted, when we wanted and that was that. During adolescence and puberty, we noticed more and more confinements and judgements being made about us, and we became more uncertain about what to do and how we would be perceived. As adults, in many ways, we would benefit by going backwards: we must keep our inner child (to a certain degree) as it mitigates many faulty fears. The older we become, we seem to want acceptance from more and more people (in our jobs, personal lives, dating and socialising), and we begin to limit our experiences, and what we can share or do in front of others. We lose our childlike and carefree attitude for fear of offending, or being seen as weak in another's eyes. Does this constricted mentality reduce our confidence? Of course it does. The more we feel like we can be ourselves, the more confident and outgoing we become and vice versa. If we ever get shy or embarrassed in front of others, it is because we feel like we have to put on a certain register, or that we cannot say and do the sort of things we would if with close friends and family. The more confident we are, the more we can do the things that will support our healthy lifestyles.

During our daily interactions, we may have a tendency to think doubtfully: "I can't believe I said that," or "How did he or she interpret what I said?" Instead, learn to simply accept whatever happened, and remain fully focused on what you think and feel about yourself. A powerful affirmation I like to use in these instances is to remind myself that neither I, nor they, will live forever, so why should I let something really get to me? This allows us to detach ourselves from the experience, and stay in the state we wish. We must learn to let go of our judgements, and what we expect others to be like. There is no need to judge or label, and do not expect that others will judge either as this can influence how we engage with others or choose not to engage with them. A general perception I have found to work is to double your positive beliefs in every situation. For example, if you are in a meeting, and you feel as though you want to say something, but you are unsure, then simply double your positivity, and how you perceive the quality of your potential response. If you are thinking, "I have quite an obvious answer, so I doubt anyone will want to hear it," then at that moment, simply think to yourself, "It is a relevant, beneficial and valid answer that they deserve to hear." The primitive brain will often belittle our notions in an attempt to keep us safe, but this is counterproductive because we will need to be expressive and opinionated in order to thrive in our careers or businesses etc. See if you can cultivate this belief in all interactions.

We all have our purpose in life. We all have our own path. We all have our own obstacles and challenges. Some inherit copious money; others live in impoverished areas; many grow up taught to be dependent; others learn that you can only count on yourself; some people lose their parents at a young age; some grow up in a hostile environment while others' parents divorce and separate the family; some *choose* to live happily while others *choose* to be a victim; some children are brought up religiously; other children are abused; many travel and experience vast cultures while others have never left their city; some grow up with disabilities while others have no ailments yet are angry. Every single person is different. We learn to judge others. We are quick to blame, and become defensive when we are blamed, but if we were to just accept and forgive people for their problems (again to an extent of course), then maybe, just maybe, we would be able to accept ourselves more. We must also learn to accept ourselves for who we are, and provide endless positivity, which should positively enhance our physiques.

All labels have limitations, even ones that appear positive. We can be labelled everywhere we go, and we learn to act accordingly to these labels. This is how we begin to form our identity and intrinsic beliefs about who we are, and what we are capable or incapable of doing. Whenever someone says or infers that you cannot do something, continue to be respectful, but make a point to either lose contact with this person or simply do not express anything meaningful with them, as they must clearly not be part of your 'troop.' We are told what we are by everyone in many different ways whether directly or indirectly. An example of a direct attack could be, "You are not very social are you?" whereas an indirect example would be, "You'll love it there because it will just be us there." Indirect presuppositions or assumptions are more likely to be accepted subconsciously by us, so be perceptive with what people may infer about you, and be wise about what you wish to accept. Everyone loves the fat, bubbly person, but that does not mean you have to be that way in order to be liked.

When we begin to simply listen to others, then we become sheep. We become followers. We give control and power to others to dictate our beliefs about our identities and thus ourselves. We lose control of our own lives, and we give others the power to shape and determine who they want us to be. Know your strengths, know what you like, know your potential, and detach from anyone else's perceptions of you especially if they are restrictive. The most important thing to take away here is to accept that judgements will be made, but keep these judgements from affecting how we think, feel and act. When we judge someone, we claim superiority. Once we understand that we all have different strengths and skills, and that we all lead different lives, then we learn not to judge or at least hold onto initial judgements. Judgements mean there is an absence of love and acceptance; displaying insufficient love means that we are fearful: to judge means to fear.

Self-Sabotage

"Resistance by definition is self-sabotage." - Steven Pressfield

Many people obtrusively entertain self-sabotaging behaviours more than they may think. Self-sabotage can be as mild as quitting a healthy-eating plan just when we are about to notice significant physical and mental improvements, or when we randomly instigate a night out that we know will involve consuming copious calories. What are your underlying beliefs about your ability to cultivate the things you desire? Some people believe the following: "I am too busy raising my children to even think about my physique." "I am spiritual being, and so I am not overly bothered with my physical appearance." These negative connotations can swirl around our subconscious, making all our decisions without us even knowing.

As we have way too much on our plates (hopefully only metaphorically speaking), we often function on autopilot, and this is when the subconscious runs amuck, unless it has been conditioned to think positively and optimistically. Our deepest fears and self-sabotaging beliefs manifest. We question things continuously: "Why do I always feel this way when this happens?" "Why do I always question myself in these situations?" These thoughts are inevitable, and to an extent, necessary. People often fail to push forward in life because they fear that they will not make it. If we feel unworthy of something, then we will wittingly or unwittingly create ways to ruin the opportunity. We will say or do something out of character, and inevitably destroy the chance we had to break through. Unfortunately, like quicksand, once we are in, and we try to force ourselves out, it is easier to get sucked in deeper and deeper until we are engulfed in debilitating actions.

"The ego mind both professes its desire for love and does everything possible to repel it, or if it gets here anyway, to sabotage it. That is why dealing with issues like control, anger and neediness is the most important work in preparing ourselves for love." – Marianne Williamson

Interestingly, the more important and challenging moments in the day are not when we are most active, but during moments of rest and silence. We are truly tested during moments of boredom. Why? Firstly, moments of boredom should be very brief; our lives should be so inundated with challenge, personal development and quality time with friends and family that we should rarely ever be bored! Frequent bouts of boredom are signs that we must change our lifestyles. We must embed better quality routines. Secondly, moments of boredom or silence are great opportunities to be appreciative, to self-reflect and to explore our goals.

Renowned scientist, Blaise Pascal explained that, "All man's miseries derive from not being able to sit quietly in a room alone." Sitting in silence mitigates all obstructions, distractions and, thus, detractions; we slow down our movements, thoughts and feelings to better access our inner workings and discover solutions. The more we move, the more we feel; the less we move, the more we think. The mind never at rest is the mind that stays in the rat race, unable to find more efficient and productive ways of living. Fascinatingly, French musician, Claude Debussy, claims that, "Music is the space between the notes." Therefore, the beauty within the music is not in the sounds, but in the silence. Our more prodigious actions are not when growing most and succeeding; it is in our inaction where we can work on the invisible, and, thus, influence the visible much more vigorously. In many ways, if we want to do more, we need to physically do less. If we want to change more, then we must give ourselves the space to mentally manoeuvre. Unfortunately, many people sabotage themselves without knowing. They inundate their lives with chaos and distractions, and fall into unnecessary traps when all they needed to do is reflect and ponder over their circumstance. If they do mentally learn something beneficial, they do not provide the mental and physical space to put it into practice. Knowledge itself is not power; knowledge comes from learning something, and then living it!

If we are to grow and become self-actualised, then we must test our characters. We must test the beliefs we have, whether these beliefs are positive or negative, so that we can find the truth. Think of a skill that you possess. Whenever you need to exhibit this proficiency, how do you test yourself? Do you play against as easier, less skilful opponent, or do you choose to face someone equally or better equipped than you? People often choose the first option because it provides them with greater certainty as they are more likely to succeed, but they will not grow if they do so. We must struggle if we are to take our aptitudes to the next level. The same applies to our fat-loss goals. We must learn to become comfortable in the uncomfortable. We must continue to push the boundaries because that is when we learn our true potential.

"The ultimate measure of a man is not where he stands in moments of comfort and convenience, but where he stands at times of challenge and controversy." - Martin Luther King Jr.

How do you react in times of adversity? Adversity builds character and resolve. Many people look for the easy way out. They go through life looking to win only if it is easy. This creates weak, short-term thinking. It creates a weak defence, and so these individuals break when they encounter struggle and challenge. They will find a way to lose, and they will mentally capitulate. Everyone can be the hammer, but not many can be the nail. They have not practiced at the highest level; they have not conditioned their minds to function supportively when things are not going according to plan. Their egos will not allow them to fully be tested and risk being wrong. Instead they will say things like, "It is all right if it doesn't work out." "My team let me down, not me." "No one helps me, so I might as well leave it." Until we take responsibility, and see what we are made of, then we cannot even begin to make the necessary changes to generate abundance in our lives. We are truly tested in moments of mental and/or physical exhaustion. Winners always find a way to win, even if they are not at their best… We learn what we are made of when in difficult situations, and when we then have the easy opportunity to quit and ruin our healthy-eating (unless this unhealthy meal was planned in advance: a cheat meal).

What do you say to yourself in moments of adversity and struggle? If you are losing in a sport, what goes through your mind? "It is too late now, we have fallen behind," or . do you say, "this is fine, I am going to build momentum and come back." These are key moments when you really learn who you are. When you play a team sport, ensure that the opposition has the better team. It is fine to 'fail.' In fact, I will use the analogy of failure in weight lifting: if you do not reach a point where you 'fail,' (cannot lift another inch) then your muscle will not grow. You need to lift until another rep cannot be completed. That is when you know you have given your all. This is how you know that you are progressing because you are going to reach the very end of your boundaries, and you are still pushing. This relentless attitude, the warrior's attitude, needs to be just as strong when it comes to eating healthily as well as when training.

Jealousy

"Always dream and shoot higher than you know you can do. Do not bother just to be better than your contemporaries or predecessors. Try to be better than yourself." – William Faulkner

Jealousy is massively futile and injurious. If we are jealous of other people's bodies, then we will never be able to create the kind of bodies we want. Do other people's successes inspire you or debilitate you? What do you think about yourself and your future? Jealousy occurs when we attach emotion to negative beliefs about what we cannot or will not accomplish. We all experience initial jealous thoughts at times, but what is important is our ability to remain detached from these thoughts. Subsequently, we must think positively about the other person's successes, consider our own potential, and attach emotion (energy) to these more beneficial thoughts. We must steer clear of jealous people. Their negativity can only detract from our successes whether they mean it or not. If someone is jealous, then they are unhelpful. Therefore, surround yourself with people who belong in your troop. The rope never runs out for some people: some want to just take and take, pull and pull, and unfortunately these people will never actually be happy. The more they take, without effort (actually doing something about their situation), the less they have. Where there is power, there is a struggle. We do not need others to influence our goals and desires.

"Loneliness does not come from having no people around you, but from being unable to communicate the things that seem most important to you." - Carl Jung

It is always beneficial to express our ideas and feelings. We must never bottle them up – it will manifest itself somehow in one form or another. Possibly, many serious illnesses derive from rigidity, and from being unable to express our inner thoughts and emotions appropriately with ourselves as well as others. This disharmony within induces illnesses. Ensuring that there is congruency amongst our thoughts, emotions and actions primarily attains mental and physical health. No one will be able to live happily and healthily if they have certain thoughts which give rise to certain emotions, but which is often suppressed for one reason or another. We must know ourselves, how we operate and provide opportunities to express our personalities appropriately. This harmony within will massively support our fat-loss endeavours, as disharmony within creates additional stress, which appears in one way or another in the form of weight gain.

Moreover, some people innately find themselves jealous. It is the state that they have become accustomed with, and it is where they return (their emotional home). Money will only make you more of what you already are. Alcohol will only make you behave how you really are or want to behave. The truth always rises to the surface. We can fake things for a moment, but no one can ever fake it for their entire lives. This is how people suppress their desires until they eventually do something awful. Acquiring more will not make us less jealous; it will just make us more jealous of people who are at the next level. Jealous people must attack it from the source: the roots of their emotional tree (what experiences have made them feel inadequate, and have ruined their self-esteem).

We can still be in good physical shape if we have powerful, yet harmful emotional homes: anger, jealousy, anxiety etc. These people use these deleterious emotional homes to perform at their best. For them it induces such emotional intensity that it gives them the energy to take action. Unfortunately for them, these painful emotional homes will never lead them to the top: true happiness. Having an emotional home of joy, peace or gratefulness will enable us to access our utmost best, and live a life of fewer afflictions. It will allow us to reach the fruit of our trees. The aim is to not have any enemies. If we are bitter or angry with someone, then these emotional connections will create chains and restrictions in other avenues. Instead we must free our souls, and unlock our true potential. The more peace we have, the more we can do freely and attract positivity, which does wonders for our physical goals.

Moving away from Fear

If we 'fail' at something, then it does not mean we are failures. If we lose at something, then we are not losers, and vice versa. A winner in life manages to sustain happiness for long periods of time whilst creating time for all types of flow-inducing activities: family time and subjective interests etc. Someone who spreads joy and knowledge creates an energy field that is impregnable, virtuous and, ultimately, undeniable. What does failure really mean? We have all 'failed' at something. Does this mean that we are all unworthy? Then what is success? If success applied everywhere, then would success even mean success as we define it? There is a yin and yang to this world: we all need to experience something painful in order to know peace. In order to have a winner, there must be a loser. In order for death to exist, there must be life. In order to have light, there must be darkness. Without discomfort, we cannot appreciate laughter. However, we must be careful not to create unnecessary pain in our lives. Instead of pain, we want to experience challenge. The more challenging our lives are, the richer our lives will become. The richer our lives become, the more energy we have, and the more we want to look after our health by eating healthily often and training often.

Discomfort teaches us that we must attack that source of discomfort one way or another. We must do the things we least want to do. We must overcome the fears that hold us back because they are never as bad as we think. Comfort teaches us the need to change our situations. When we are uncomfortable, we must seek comfort (by improving upon our weakness), and when we are comfortable, we must seek discomfort (push ourselves and continually grow). This continuous cycle results in successful accomplishments. It is all about pushing our boundaries even if we currently feel successful and happy. There is always more we can learn. There is always more we can give. There is always more we can create. We must seek discomfort. This is why many of our daily routines must be uncomfortable: we want to remain disciplined, and to build our mental and emotional stamina.

Life incessantly tests us. It throws challenges upon us to see how we react: not getting the grade we wanted, arguments with friends, losing a loved one and so on. Be like water: be flexible; flow naturally; be yourself; give life (energy). Unfortunately, many people design their own misfortune, wittingly or unwittingly, and they can be created for different purposes (often procrastination, avoiding boredom perilously, having something to talk about and becoming the victim as a way of blaming others for our dire state). If we lived forever, we all know that life would become lacklustre. Phrases like carpe diem and live for the moment would not exist because we can always live another moment infinitely. This is why we must maximise our potential, and live this way for as long as we can. Make the necessary changes now. Failing can be highly beneficial or devastating depending on our conditioning. If we value what others think about us above our quest for inner and outer success, then we have lost on the biggest scale. If we do not fail, then we are true failures in life itself. We therefore failed on the largest scale of all: we failed ourselves.

"You might never fail on the scale I did, but some failure in life is inevitable. It is impossible to live without failing at something, unless you live so cautiously that you might as well not have lived at all – in which case, you fail by default." –
J.K. Rowling

Signs

"The past speaks to us in a thousand voices, warning and comforting, animating and stirring to action." – Felix Adler

Our egos are our biggest enemy as they can blind us from seeing what we need to see. Everything happens for a reason. Life's nudges are always asking if we are ready to learn, change and grow. Let us look at an example where something horrible had a beneficial lesson: I once had an awful chest infection. One of the symptoms and consequences of chest infections is that your appetite is significantly suppressed (this will be important shortly). Obviously, I was bedridden, and so I had no option but to watch the television (something I am not a proponent of generally). Over time, I had accumulated many unseen movies that I intended on watching. One was a movie about Mahatma Ghandi. While I was watching the movie, there was a scene where Ghandi would fast as part of his philosophy regarding non-violence. Whilst watching, I thought to myself, "I wonder if fasting would benefit my current situation since my body is naturally telling me not to eat." I would usually force myself to eat during colds because I believed that it would increase energy and recovery. However, I learned that when eating solid foods, our digestive systems work hard to digest and assimilate these foods, and so I became intrigued.

After researching the usefulness of fasting, I somehow found my way onto YouTube videos that elicited the benefits of intermittent fasting. My curiosity propelled me to read various books and listen to various audio books alike that exclaimed the usefulness of intermittent and full-day fasting. After incorporating these strategies into my health regime, I felt lighter, more energetic and sharper, and my body has never looked or felt so good. The moral of the story is simple: all things guide us down the path that we truly want or need. Our unconscious desires create circumstances and events that manifest our reality. Unfortunately, many people do not recognise the signs in their lives where they can change their thoughts and feelings about something. This is mostly due to being unchangeable due to fear, stubbornness/ignorance and losing control. Sometimes 'bad' things must happen for better things to come.

There are signs and signals all around us. The universe is constantly communicating with us. A physical injury tried to teach someone something: maybe it is to slow down, or maybe it is a physical manifestation of negative thinking, an accumulation of fearful and anxious thoughts that imploded indirectly. Maybe it is that we must focus more on our minds rather than perpetually living purely in the physical and active world. Alternatively, that minor car accident could be the most important thing to ever happen to a person: it may have prevented them from experiencing a far more fatal car accident later in life. It may have foreshadowed an ominous danger that someone fortunately and hopefully learned from. That missed job opportunity could be a godsend; a person may have found his or her way into a totally different and far more rewarding profession as a result. That breakup that felt so devastating may be a wonderful separation: a person may have realised that his or her partner held them back in many ways, and now this individual has the time and energy to pursue something far more worthwhile (emotionally and/or financially). These are life's signs that we must change. If we do not observe them, and do something about them, then greater afflictions are forthcoming. We get so immersed and absorbed in our own lives that we cannot notice the holes we will soon fall into. These are signs and opportunities for us to reflect on our lives up until now, and evaluate how we can move forward. Every event has its purpose. If we cannot see it, we are not stepping back enough. Take a step back, check our egos, slow down our processes, and objectively make the changes needed. The more we reduce pain, the easier it is to stay on the right path, and ultimately develop the kind of body that makes us proud.

It is immensely significant to address and tackle issues sooner than later. When we notice a subtle issue in something we think, feel, do or see in others, then we attack the issue then and there. Whether it is by subtly and empathetically let someone know that a behaviour was wrong, or directly doing whatever we want to resolve the issue, we must kill it while it is small. Leaving things because they are 'small' is precarious and unwise. Never underestimate the opponent due to its current size. Think long term and imagine the kind of monster that it can turn into if we arrogantly allow it to do so. All things start small. We want to prevent its escalation by improving communication with others and ourselves.

What makes people change their lifestyles? Unfortunately, many people have to experience life threatening or devastating consequences for them to make a change. Life will throw many incrementally and progressively painful signs our way until we learn from our mistakes and sometimes not even then! For instance, if a person is always very frantic in the morning, doing many things hurriedly, and then leaves a tap running by accident, then that is a small sign that they must have a calmer start to the day. On another occasion, if the same person is excessively rushing through things, and then on the way out of the house, leaves the front door open by accident, then that is another sign. One day, this person will forgetfully leave the cooker on, and accidentally burn the house down. Why? They never listened to and reacted to the smaller signs! Others, fortunately, do not wait. Instead, they always want to push forward obstinately, always improving and appreciating that they will never become happy, as they *are* happiness itself. Happiness is incessant progression in any avenue that holds significance. The happier we are, the more we want to take care of our bodies and ourselves.

"While it may seem small, the ripple effects of small things is extraordinary." – Matt Bevin

The Negative Voice

"Learn to forgive others so that you can release yourself from being held captive by the very negative thoughts around you." – Stephen Richards

The quotation above also relates to how we forgive and accept ourselves as a way of releasing the shackles of negativity that prevent us from truly living abundantly. We can never demolish our negative voice, but we can learn to calm it down, and to question its cogency. The more we question something, the weaker it becomes, and the more it loses its validity. We must question this diminishing puppet whenever we experience a negative or limiting thought. We must question all of our negative thoughts and feelings, but we must learn not to question our positive thoughts and certainties regarding our aptitude. Perceive a positive action as being a brick that we will add one on top of the other to create our mansion of joy. This is necessary if we are to provide the mind and body with the energy required to consistently make the right choices for our health and physiques.

Our intrinsic negative voices are not really us. It is often the part of our brains that attempts to compromise our success. It can take many forms. It is our self-doubt. It is our feelings of inadequacy. It is the masochist within that relishes in our misfortune, or the sadist that enjoys the difficulties that others face. The negative voice questions our actions; it is the voice that forces us to remain inert. Have you ever convinced yourself to give something up, or to do something that you knew was deleterious? Think of a goal you had or still have that you have not achieved yet. How did it fall apart? How long did it take to dissipate? What did you say to yourself? What obstacles intervened? How did you present this failure to yourself?

Here are some prevalent, common things we would expect to hear from the negative voice: "Why are you even going to bother trying to lose fat when you can just accept that you're incapable of keeping it off?" "You will never be disciplined enough to lose fat because you have always given in to your urges." "You are pushing yourself a bit too hard in the gym. Remember we have other things to do today. What's the point anyway?" The negative voice knows your weaknesses, and it zooms in on them. It is like a professional, personal bully that we have to deal with for the rest of our lives. We have to learn to calm the bully down by making it less insecure, giving it metaphorical hugs and showing it affection whilst rarely listening to it of course.

Accept that this voice, to some extent, is impossible to eradicate. The divinity within must flourish and overwhelm in order for us to live abundantly and with clarity. What type of things can we say to appease our built-in negativity? "I deserve to be happy." "I am going to instill a healthy habit every single month, so that I can lose the weight and keep it off." "I am so grateful for everything that I have. Any more is just a bonus that I will make the most of." "What current strengths do I have that can help me to lose weight and live healthily?" The problem people may have with accepting this notion is that they confuse their logical human mind with arrogance, and so suppress the light that should be allowed to spread. Some people think that loving themselves is narcissistic and repulsive, but if we do not love ourselves, then how can we ever attract the quality things that we all deserve? In writing this book, I had so many internal battles, at different stages, regarding a whole host of different aspects. This book in itself exemplifies how our human, loving side can, and should, influence the negative side.

Giving up is easy, but resilience takes effort and energy. Whatever is hard to achieve is always more valuable. We need to get used to seeing things through to the end. It is crucial to persist when facing negativity or self-repudiation. We might have an idea (say to start exercising every morning), and then, over time, if not initially, we begin to allow negative suggestions to intrude and impede upon our dreams: "Oh don't be daft, you will not be able to always wake up at that time and get to work. I mean it will be cold on some days. Sometimes the day will be too busy." This limiting belief will soon seep its way into our reality unless we have strong affirmations and incantations in place to keep us moving forward. Life works like a seesaw. Think of your brain as the stable part in the middle of the seesaw. You now have two sides that swing back and forth: the positive voice and the negative voice. The side that wins will be the side that has more weight: more affirmations, energy and momentum (a stronger emotional charge). It is your seesaw after all, so why not choose its constituents? If it is your playground, then play it by your rules. Create a list of life rules and principles that you promise to adhere to from here on out. As long as you keep doing these things, then you will always have a good body at the very least even if other things take precedence in your life at different stages, which is only natural.

Limiting Beliefs

"Whatever you hold in your mind on a consistent basis is exactly what you will experience in your life." - Tony Robbins

Until we work on our beliefs, especially our limiting beliefs, then we will massively struggle to attract what we want in our lives. We must work on eliminating our limiting beliefs. Firstly, what is a belief? A belief occurs when we feel absolutely certain about something. What is a limiting belief? It is a way of thinking that prohibits us from developing in an area. We therefore feel absolutely certain that we cannot overcome certain things. Here are some general limiting beliefs to help us to identify our own underlying limiting beliefs: "I can't get a degree because no one in my family has ever got one." "I can't learn about stocks because I am not good with charts and numbers." "Hats do not suit me." These are signs of having a fixed mindset: we do not believe we can make progress, as we believe skills are purely natural. This then becomes a self-fulfilling prophecy. Carol Dweck teaches the importance of having a growth mindset: being open minded, and believing that we can improve regardless of our current aptitudes.

We all have negative beliefs, some of which we are aware of and others we are completely oblivious. These assumptions do not help at all, and in many ways, the more we question these things, the less certainty and confidence we have in our capacities. It is detrimental and immobilising to ever say that we cannot achieve something. Considering that something can be attained creates the possibility for creativity, and the drive necessary to take action. However, saying something will never happen, for whatever reason, drives this affirmation into a stable belief system, a negative paradigm, that can even have a knock-on-effect on other things that we 'cannot' do. We must believe that we can dictate our physical appearance by being able to control our thoughts, feelings and actions. People whose weight fluctuates randomly are usually those who have things dictated to them in their lives. They are moulded the way others have chosen indirectly. If you have a great body consistently, then it is a sign that you are in control of your life and your destiny.

"The only differences between people who think they are creative and people who think they are not are their beliefs about their creativity. Start telling yourself that you are a creative person." - **Sanaya Roman**

We must always question the negative thoughts that we have, but never question when we are confident and certain. Examples of how to question negative thoughts are as follows: "Should I always be so harsh on myself?" "Is it healthy to oppress my true feelings?" Only question these things IF we have positive answers to respond with! For example, "How come I get completely stressed?" A negative answer would be: "I get stressed because I am not enough, and I am setting myself up for failure." A positive answer would be: "I get stressed because I want to present myself in the best possible light, which I can do if I just relax." Questioning our confidence and ability as it relates to our fat-loss goals can have an adverse effect. Here are some examples: "Am I really capable of losing all that weight?" "Will I be able to perform like that again?" "Is my emotional intelligence strong enough to lose and keep the weight off?" The more we question positive thoughts, the less certain and confident we become. Instead, we want to question our negative thoughts, so that these debilitating thoughts become less and less impervious.

How can we change our limiting beliefs? Have you ever thought you could not achieve something (a job promotion, being able to fit into a certain outfit, being in a relationship with a great person), and then one day you did? You now know this is possible. We all encounter negative, limiting beliefs, but we must understand that this fearful side is a primitive part of our brain, and that it is not actually our own thoughts! Furthermore, we have a 'human' part within our brain, and this puts things into perspective. It is loving and logical. Unfortunately, according to Steve Peters, the primitive part of our brain is five times more powerful than our human side! Therefore, it is down to us to condition our brains to ensure that we know when the primitive brain is hijacking us, and to know when, and how, to emphasise the human whenever the 'chimp' comes out. This takes practice, so be patient. Here is an example: You are contemplating what you should eat for your next meal. Below is your inner dialogue (your human brain (HB), and your primitive brain (PB)):

PB: "I have to eat right now! I am starving."

HB: "I am going to make a salad quickly."

PB: "Don't even bother. It takes too much time. Just eat! Just order a takeaway."

HB: "That will set me back massively. I need to eat a salad, so that I can feel light. I've got too much work to do."

PB: "A salad won't be enough. Will a burger and chips really set you back that much?"

HB: "Yes. If I give in today, then I cannot trust myself tomorrow. I cannot show weakness. I must be strong."

PB: "You are taking all this healthy eating stuff way too seriously. Are you going to live forever or something?"

HB: "Why should I ruin my healthy eating if I do not have to? I am in control."

PB: "It is only a matter of time until this stupid diet is over! Let us be honest"

HB: "I will really respect myself for going for what I want in life. I want to feel strong, healthy and sexy. I need to be consistent if I am to succeed in all avenues."

In this instance, the HB does a great job with calming the 'chimp.' We can never eliminate our primitive thoughts, but we can learn to dance with it and appease the PB. The most important thing is to cut this conflicting inner dialogue short to prevent ourselves from overthinking: paralysis by analysis. Take action. Our minds often work on autopilot. This is when the subconscious takes over. This is where learned thoughts, feelings and routines circulate, and continue our underlying belief systems. The mind is left to wander, and it reverts to what it knows (our default mode), where it is comfortable, and that is where our deep desires and fears live. These can definitely be changed if we are self-reflective, persistent and catch ourselves when the mind falls into the same traps.

People believe that for one thing to get better in life, something else has to fall back. This is untrue. Yes, to reach a high level of achievement in any endeavour requires great focus, dedication and sacrifice, but this does not mean something else has to cave in. That in itself is a limiting belief. Instead, perceive things as working synergistically: it is about improving our self-esteem. Confidence means feeling competence at a given activity. However, self-esteem refers to how we respect and love ourselves, and thus partake in challenging activities with more self-appreciation. The stronger our self-esteem, the more we are likely to put ourselves out there, and really go for what we want. If we want a leaner and more muscular body, then we must value ourselves and devote effort and energy into our bodies.

Obsessions and Addictions

"Every form of addiction is bad, no matter whether the narcotic be alcohol, morphine or idealism." – Carl Jung

There is a thin line between magnificence and madness. An obsession can be both incredibly beneficial yet incredibly destructive. We all have obsessions and addictions. It is down to us to choose those that are positive and beneficial rather than self-destructive. Negative addictions can provide instant relief, but they increase stress levels in the long run. Negative addictions might be pleasurable in the moment, but they can set us back when we stop doing them. An addiction controls us; it has leverage over us. Our addictions, even beneficial ones, will ultimately lead to our downfall. However, it is better to choose a downfall that had many amazing, pleasurable moments rather than a downfall consisting of pain and struggle throughout.

An obsession can take many different forms. An obsession occurs when we cannot take our minds off something even if we wanted to change our focus. An obsession is a mental compulsion whereas an addiction is when you are physically compelled to do things (this often incurs withdrawal symptoms when abstaining from them). If we do not change our behaviours when we know we should, then, quite simply, we have not suffered enough. It relates to the pleasure and pain principle. If there is more pain than pleasure when doing something, then we will not want to do it and vice versa. It all comes down to our perceptions of what is pleasurable and what is painful.

All obsessions and addictions, in one way or another, stem from our fears. If we fear not being attractive enough, then we become obsessed with our appearance, and so addicted to improving our looks. If we fear being lonely, then we become obsessed with being around other people, and so addicted to manifesting bad things just so we can gain sympathy from others. If we fear losing control in life, then we become obsessed with monitoring everything around us, and addicted to telling people what to do. What we fear most comes true, so why not work to change our fears? Everyone will encounter moments of struggle when improving and becoming more adept at something, so consider what you say to yourself to keep you going in moments of uncertainty. We have been programmed to always be fearful of something. This fear shifts throughout our lives depending on what we have learned to conquer. At one stage in our life we might fear losing our spouse, at another we might fear developing an illness, at another we might fear losing our looks, at another we might fear going to sleep, at another we might fear our financial futures and so on. Once we conquer one fear, then another one will appear. It is very important to understand this because when the fear changes, it is a sign that we have conquered the previous one. If we continue to fight our fear of not looking the way we want to look, then we will continue to find answers (such as learning from this book) until we erase this fear and turn it into a certainty.

An obsession originates from a set of patterns. We become so engrossed with the emotions experienced that we allow the emotions to override any rational thought. Most people know when they are obsessed, yet they cannot withdraw from thinking, feeling and acting upon it still. This is because the entire process has not been fully thought through and the root of the obsession has not been fully explored. However, the more we activate our rational brains, the more we think things through, and break down the emotions attached to this action. Once we break an obsession down into the steps that we take mentally and emotionally until we complete the action, then it is much easier to intervene. An obsession also becomes less powerful once we break it down because we have taken some of the variety and excitement away: we know the process that we are going through, which takes away some of the impulsivity, therefore making the process more mundane and less gripping. Extract all of the reasons why we do whatever it is that we do. Then we can naturally dissipate the emotions involved, and it is precisely the emotion that drives us to act upon our compulsions. These emotions strengthen over time, and the more we take part in the activity, the more we naturally want to push the boundaries more and more. Doing too much of anything is dangerous. Our obsession will lead to our downfall if not managed properly.

There is a difference between being driven, and being unable to stop ourselves from doing something. Motivation and inspiration are pleasant whereas obsessions uncontrollably weaken our very sense of self. Our obsessions and addictions create mental chaos.

These addictions make us lose trust in ourselves. This mistrust pervasively affects how we think about our competence in other areas too such as our discipline, focus and beliefs around healthy eating and exercising. We must ensure that our obsessions are geared towards supporting our health, and that our addictions take us closer to our fat-loss goals.

Chapter 4: Psychology – Simplicity

"There is no greatness where there is no simplicity, goodness and truth." – Leo Tolstoy

We must create simplicity in our lives at every opportunity. Most people think that more is better. They believe that if things are complex, then they must be good. This is not only wrong, but it can be quite damaging. Think about the things you have to do every day: organising things, fixing or cleaning things, travelling, eating, conversing, meetings, social media and so on. The more complex we make all of these things, the more stressful our lives become. We want to make things as simple and efficient as possible, and some things we will want to delegate or eradicate if they are classed as menial. Complexity induces stress, and this stress compounds over the course of the day, resulting in unhealthy food choices as a way of providing short-term immediate gratification. The more stressed and unhappy we are with what we do every day, the more prone we are to seeking short-term pleasures that are really no good for us in the long term. Leaders are long-term thinkers; followers are short-term thinkers. If you want to create, and sustain, the kind of body you want, then you have to lead your life on your terms. We may have to find more fulfilling careers in order to change our perceptions, joy and health. We may have to change our relationships if we are to condition our minds better. We might even have to change where we live in order to feel safer, happier and less stressed. Simplicity induces peace. Peace induces clarity. Clarity induces consistency. Consistency induces quality results.

Simple Mindset

"Mind is a flexible mirror, adjust it, to see a better world." – Amit Ray

The unexpected will arrive when we are unprepared. If we have made life simple for ourselves (by deciding upon things more quickly, reducing drama, reducing how many urgent things we must do etc.), then we will be well equipped to handle the wonderful or horrendous surprises that are inevitable. The issues most individuals have is that they become so self-absorbed and involved in the 'rat-race,' that they develop what I call the 'inadequacy syndrome' or 'progression complex.' We get too drawn into the game of doing 'better' than others within our fields, that we lose touch with the bigger focus: abundance in all avenues. We also lose touch with what is fundamentally important and natural: kindness, giving and acceptance. We judge and criticise ourselves, and others, based on questionable means.

When people are caught off guard, it is easier for them to lose their discipline. Unforeseen challenges in our personal and professional lives can challenge our discipline and daily structure. They will eat and drink the things that they did not plan. Their routines can be muddled. This is how some people fall off the horse. Once they fall off, it can be harder to get back on the right path unless they have conditioned themselves to eat well and train well for a long time. The more proactive we are in all areas, the less likely, or less often, we are going be caught unexpectedly, and so we can remain consistent with our healthy routines and ways of thinking. It is not just about losing one's composure; what is even more important is how quickly we can recover, and get back on the right path.

Live a beautiful life by not being attached to anything. There is no need to fully belong to a specific friendship group, cult or organisation. We do not have to pick one thing, and elicit hatred for anything different. We are complex and beautiful beings. We may love to read, yet love to practice martial arts. We may love to speak philosophy and psychology, yet love to listen to silly and crude stand-up comedy. We may value silence, and recognise its therapeutic effects, yet value socialising. Things are not black and white. This flexibility in our mindset will enable us to react well to most situations. It ensures that we do not label ourselves, and thus limit ourselves. The simple and flexible mindset is to believe that we can excel in many diverse areas of life. Yes, we can live amazing healthy lifestyles whilst being talented in other areas. Unfortunately, others are more rigid in their beliefs. We do not have to believe that we must choose a select few things, and label ourselves and others based on these alone. We must appreciate our diverse nature and interests. It keeps us balanced. We should love all that we do, yet remain separated from such things, and still be exhilarated and active. For example, it is about being absolutely devoted to being lean and feeling strong whilst not needing to be so. The more we need many things, the more egotistical we become. Being indefinable is a sensational feeling. We can feel emancipated to take up any activity, and feel as though we can both belong to it and can learn from its teachings. This growth mindset will keep us driven and thus happy throughout our lives, enabling us to make better decisions regarding our health.

There is a clear connection between our inner and outer worlds. They go hand in hand in many ways. If we want a clearer mind, then we should clear and organise our physical space whether that be our offices, our bedrooms, our homes etc. Physical clutter creates mental clutter and vice versa. We should clear out what we do not need, and replace old, archaic things with newer more useful things and information. If we want to change our lives, then we must change our surroundings. The more we have, the more complicated and stressed our minds function. We tend to make worse decisions that will negatively affect our fat-loss desires if we are stressed. There is a reason why Steve Jobs wore the same outfit every day. Look at everything we do, and we should ask ourselves, how can we make this simpler? Simplicity induces clarity and focus. Ironically enough, the easiest options can give us the best results. Many people think that the more they acquire, the happier they will be; they hoard what they have, and keep adding to the pile, inadvertently and unwittingly creating their future struggles. They limit the options available, and consequently derail and hinder progress. Why? We become so inundated with what we perceive to be good (excessive belongings) that we indirectly begin to teach ourselves that more is better. This belief spreads across many areas including our relationships with food. We become restricted in our ability to move forward because we fear what we might lose.

Concentrate on quality over quantity. Focus on acquiring beautiful and meaningful possessions that we will use frequently as opposed to purchasing overwhelmingly copious things that clutters space and thus our minds. This is why people naturally love ceilings that are high up, as well as large open spaces, as they condition the mind to think more openly and abundantly. The sky is the limit. We become like our private environments. Moreover, many people inundate their lives with endless, often unimportant tasks, and this kills our energy levels. The lower our energy levels, the more susceptible we are ' to eat and drink unhealthily. We all react to stress in our own ways. We must ensure that we detach ourselves from things in order to make better choices for our health. A lack of patience, along with the consequent shorter temper, has made it harder than ever to simply sit in silence and think in solitude. This lack of being with oneself in the truest sense has led us to be tenser and disconnected within. This obviously hinders how we function in the world, and thus it becomes easier to lose our discipline and focus. Only when the mind is silent will the muse be more likely to show. Only when the mind is quiet can we experience flow and clarity. We need flow and clarity to enjoy life more. We must enjoy life more in order to have strong self-esteem. We need strong self-esteem to follow our passions such as developing the kind of body that fulfils us.

A clogged up mind will choke and fail to rise to the occasion. Abstain from taking in nonsensical and futile information. Conceive a plastic bag as a metaphor for our minds. The more we put inside a 'bag,' the more pressure and tension (stress) we add. If we fill the bag too much, then it will rip and capitulate. One of the limiting beliefs people have is that life is hard and complicated. We could make our lives as complicated and busy as we want, but that may not lead to success in any department. Simplifying where possible ensures that we have the energy, instinctive brilliance and wherewithal to rise to the occasion when something truly challenging arrives. This is how simplicity creates abundance. The noisiest people, things and lives often hold the least strength and power. As the saying goes, the emptiest can makes the most noise. Claude Debussy fascinatingly expressed that, "Music is the silence between the notes." View the notes as being what our senses experience (our external world), and view the silence between the notes as being our inner world. If we want to consistently eat healthily and train well, then we must make things simpler; we must have clarity and reduce unnecessary emotional responses to things, which happen when we have too many unhelpful things swirling in our minds.

Variety

"Variety's the very spice of life, that gives it all its flavor."
– William Cowper

Tony Robbins teaches that we have a need for certainty and control in life, yet we also have a need for variety in order to keep us mentally and emotionally stimulated. It is down to us to seek variety in supportive ways rather than giving into life's more destructive variants. Where there is variety there is choice. The more choices we have, the more we can choose supportive outcomes and vice versa. However, the more choices we have, the harder it can be to make the right choice also. Think about the ways in which you experience variety in life. Consider which of these supports the quality of your life, and which ones weaken your spirit. We must replace unsupportive habits with more empowering ones.

People who have addictive personalities tend to require a great deal of variety. They become bored very easily, and regularly require having their adrenaline and senses stimulated. If we know ourselves, then it becomes easier to channel our energy in the right areas. We can plan when to be creative, and when to take risks, such as by going to certain places or partaking in exciting activities. We must be able to plan when we can experience variety otherwise it will be arbitrary. If we allow ourselves to be random with our need for variety, then we will often choose to be random, not only more often, but also at the easiest times. If we condition ourselves to be impulsive whenever we feel like being impulsive, then we risk ruining our health and fat-loss goals on a daily basis.

Our Inner Child

"Some day you will be old enough to start reading fairy tales again." – C.S. Lewis

An unconventional strategy to help us lose body-fat is to return to a more simplistic mindset in a way. We must keep the child within us alive as adults if we are to focus on what we want, and if we are to express ourselves the way we should. Over time, we have our inquisitiveness, creativity and desire to do what we want taken away from us by our elders, society and the educational system. We learn to know our roles and fit in somewhere. However, in order to thrive in life, and to create the body we want, we need to be playful, fun and do what comes naturally to us, as this increases energy and enables us to keep following our dreams: some people think it is childlike to be focused on our bodies too much. We need to remain flexible, to value ourselves and to think originally. The beauty of life is being natural. Unfortunately, this can be very challenging for some. As young children, we possess these skills. Children have a certain carelessness. They often do not care about how others perceive them; they desire complete freedom. This slowly and gradually gets taken from us. We enter the educational system where we are told exactly how to be, and we are criticised left, right and centre. The older we become, the more responsibilities we undertake; we must care for others more, and become increasingly mindful of how others perceive us. We wear suits, usually because we have to, and we learn that we must speak a certain way to appear appropriate and sophisticated, again usually to please others and fit in. We are told what we can and cannot do by our parents, siblings, teachers and elders. We become detrimentally moulded and broken down gradually until we fit into our own little box. Our dreams and desires constantly face limitations and restrictions. And so we learn to repress what we really want, which subsequently becomes engrained into our unconscious. This dying fire lays dormant. It is never too late to light the fire of freedom.

We all have an inner child. It is the part within us that just wants to laugh, be expressive, say how we really feel and chase the dreams we have. Being childlike and natural can enable us make the decisions we want to make based on our subjective desires rather than doing and being the way we are expected to be. If we do as expected, then we will become mediocre, and there are not many ordinary people who have incredible bodies. Most people have their inner child suppressed because they need to 'grow up.' They are taught in the workforce to be professional, accept things as they are and adhere to the business' cultural etiquette. Instead most people become physically and mentally rigid. They lose the spring in their step. They become accustomed to low energy, low vibrations and mediocre relationships. Are you restricted in life? How and why? How can this be changed? Why must this be changed? It comes down to how we were raised, and how people have conditioned us. Unless we are mindful, people can knowingly or unknowingly try to make us feel insufficient, and as though we are lacking in an area. It is a weak, insecure tactic to try and wield power over us, and it works on many. This is so they get what they want by making us feel insecure, but the self-actualised human being does not care for this. The self-actualised among us are never coaxed by this game, and they are fully aware that they are in charge of how they think and feel about themselves. If we believe that we *need* anything, apart from psychological, survival reasons, then we have been influenced and manipulated.

Same Meals

Eating healthily becomes a lot easier when we have an eating schedule. It removes complexity and provides stability. We know that if we eat these similar meals every day, then not only will we provide ourselves with the necessary nutrients each day, we will also reduce the amount of unplanned food we can eat each day. Pick three well-sized meals to eat each day, and ensure that you eat a range vegetables and salads each day. You may want to eat these off your plate first otherwise we have a tendency to save them for last and often when we are most full, which means that we will sometimes not want to eat them. Schedule roughly what times you want to eat these three main meals, so that you make it habitual. Planning our daily eating program in advance removes additional decision-making from our daily lives, which provides us with greater certainty. It enables us to focus more on other important things for the day such as our family, careers and so on.

Weekly Training Schedule

As with our habitual eating schedule, we will also want to plan our weekly training program. This should prevent us from overtraining whilst again simplifying our decision-making. If we know when and how we will be training, then we can adjust the intensity of our workouts depending on what we have planned for the next day.

Let us look at individual workouts. If we want to maintain our muscle mass, then we will want to lift weights initially, and then finish our workout with cardio. We can either do a whole-body weight workout where we ensure that most muscles are worked on a smaller level but every day, or we can choose certain muscle groups to blitz on certain days. This is really down to your preference. It also depends on what body parts you wish to prioritise depending on your muscular proportions. One thing is for sure, you will want to utilise compound movements more often such as squats, deadlifts and bench press. Think about what body parts you want to really develop. Train them daily and/or dedicate an entire workout for that body part often.

Simple Planning

Productive, hard-working people often create unrealistic to-do lists for each day, which invariably leaves them feeling inadequate and stressed every day. This chronic stress is hazardous to our health goals. Instead of needing to do millions of useful things every day, some of which are unimportant, we should seek to do something useful within our key areas if we are to ensure balance and pleasure. As long as we do something each day to help us achieve our priorities (our health, wealth and relationships), then we should be satisfied with how the day went. There is no need for a huge to-do list every day, as it can demoralise and reduce our self-esteem over time. This stressful daily grind can ruin our energy levels, and make us think unsatisfactorily about ourselves, thereby ruining our self-esteem and our desire to do what is best for our bodies. If we simplify what we must do each day, then we feel a greater sense of control and accomplishment. Think about your usual to-do list and think about how important it is in the grand scheme of things. What one thing can you do to enhance the quality of your main relationships? What one thing can you do today to improve your health and fat-loss goals? What one thing can you do to directly or indirectly increase your wealth?

Focus on the next Step

Whilst it is important to think long term in order to make better health-related decisions, we must also take one day at a time. As long as we always focus on our mental and emotional state in the current moment, then we will never really go off course unless we plan it (cheat meal). Keep it simple, and focus purely on the present moment. The moment we start to think that we must be disciplined for an entire day or week, then we begin to relinquish our power in the now. The ability to be present and not to think about the past or future is really important. Yes, there is a time to reflect on how an event transpired, or what our future might be like, but this kind of thinking should really take place when we are feeling mentally, emotionally and physically strong. If we feel tired, annoyed or stressed, and then we think of the past or future (as it relates to eating or training), then we will only be able to muster unsupportive reactions that usually result in making bad choices. In these moments, we must either change our state or remove ourselves from our surroundings (where there might be treats for instance).

Decisiveness

We must condition ourselves to make decisions quickly. Sometimes we might think about whether we should or should not eat an unhealthy treat several times in the same day! As a general rule, let us decide within five seconds if we wish to have our 'cheat' meal or not for the week, and we must not return to this question again later. There is no need for doubt or hesitation. The more you question something, the more it loses its power.

Here is an example:

"It has been a long day. I just want to eat something delicious and quickly, so I can just relax."

"But should I really give in? Is it necessary?"

"I will probably just eat like a pig for 10 minutes, and then regret it for the rest of the week. What's the point?"

"But I deserve it. I was awesome today."

"Maybe I should just eat half. It won't do that much damage surely."

"Half will just get the ball rolling. You will want more because that is how you always work. You never do anything halfheartedly!"

"Do I really need to punish myself like this? If I really feel like eating it, then I should."

There were several instances in the example above where there was doubt and uncertainty. The more this dialogue takes place, the more we end up giving in. We must learn to cut it short, and to be firm. This is how simple the internal dialogue should be:

"It has been a long day. I just want to eat something delicious and quickly, so I can just relax."

"You've been awesome today, and you are going to keep being strong. It's as simple as that. Go and make something healthy to eat, and then relax."

It really is as simple as that. You were firm with yourself, and you phrased things positively. You also cut the dialogue short; there were no options given to work with. It was clear. This tough love is necessary if we are to consistently make quality choices for ourselves.

We need to take responsibility, and we must not justify going off course. We can always come up for a reason as to why we faltered with our eating plans: "My partner annoyed me today, so I am going to treat myself." "I didn't sleep well last night, so I am going to treat myself." "I worked hard all day long, so I am going to treat myself." "My spouse doesn't give me the attention I want, so I am going to treat myself." "I am out with my friends, so I am going to treat myself." "My business is my priority today, so I am going to treat myself." It is easy to justify a bad action; it is hard to hold yourself accountable.

Boredom

Interestingly, the more important and challenging moments in the day are not when we are most active, but during moments of rest and silence. We are truly tested during moments of boredom. Why? Firstly, moments of boredom should be very brief; our lives should be so inundated with challenge, personal development and quality time with friends and family that we should rarely ever be bored! Frequent bouts of boredom are signs that we must change our lifestyles. We must embed better quality routines. Secondly, moments of boredom or silence are great opportunities to be appreciative, to self-reflect and to explore our goals.

People tend to eat when they are bored. Boredom is often a result of being unable to keep oneself stimulated. It often results in negative thinking and subsequent eating as a distraction. Part of living an active and healthy lifestyle is really down to how well we plan our lives. If we have clear goals, then we will always have things that we should be working on. We must block out our time every day. It is necessary to create an hourly schedule for our day. The better we plan, the less time we waste. This keeps energy and productivity high whilst eliminating excess emotions and overeating. Think about the times in the day when you are most bored. How do you fill up this time? Does it, in one way or another, affect how much you eat or what you eat? Boredom that lasts a matter of minutes is understandable. However, if boredom lasts for hours, then there is a larger issue. Perhaps we need to consider our hobbies, interests and desires. Perhaps we need to fall in love with learning and sharing ideas and skills. Boredom directly relates to lost potential.

Comparisons

Comparing ourselves to others can connote low self-esteem. We seek reassurance and self-worth by measuring ourselves against others. Jealousy itself is a sign that we compare ourselves to others also. We limit ourselves every time we compare ourselves to people. It often portrays our levels of insecurity. Anyway the more we compare ourselves to others within a given field, the less we are likely to partake in those activities. It is a sure fire way to put yourself off. This is why we must just remain focused on our own appearance and health otherwise we can lose our motivation to constantly improve. Therefore, we must condition ourselves to never compare like this. If we do compare, however, then it should only be with people who are better than us at something. When we compare ourselves with others, we lower our standards and justify doing worse. Ideally, we must only compete with our own potential in terms of the quality of how we train and eat each week. Our progress is more important than our actual results. People who are preoccupied with results will never ever be happy with how they are doing. We must instead become obsessed with the process of getting into shape. Take pleasure in the daily things you do consistently that make a small difference every single day.

Connection

One of the biggest reasons why people lose their motivation to train and eat healthily is because we often do it in isolation or with minimal connection with others. If we want to change our body composition for the long term, then we will want to base it around our most meaningful relationships where possible. We should involve others in our healthy routines. We should train with our friends and loved ones. We should eat healthily with them, and support each other's goals. We can develop a sense of connection by doing positive, healthy things with the people we love. This creates quality associations. It also makes unexciting things far more enjoyable (even though I personally have conditioned myself to enjoy the healthy routines I have instilled!). We tend to appreciate partaking in things that make us feel more connected with people. In addition, it makes us feel like we are contributing to others' lives, and that we are not being selfish by only doing things that, on the surface level, appear self-obsessed. It is also a way for us to hold each other accountable. If we begin to do healthy things together, then we not only push ourselves harder, but we can also ensure that we remain consistent. No one wants to let a loved one down when they have put on their trainers ready to go for a run. No one wants to let a loved one down when they are looking forward to cooking a great, healthy meal together. Consider the different healthy routines you want to embed, and identify when and how you can incorporate friends, family and your partner into joining you.

No Other Way

If we are to truly develop the kind of body we desire, then we must be prepared to burn our bridges. When there are options, even good ones in life, then there are dilemmas and possibilities. We want to remove all other possibilities. One way is to give away all our oversized, or undersized, clothes – or the clothes that we no longer wish to fit in – even if they are expensive! We must make a statement. We must be willing to give away our invested money and resources if they, in any form, support our old unhealthy ways. It is literally a matter of choosing to be overweight yet fit into all the expensive clothes we have bought, or choose the ideal body we want. We may want to put on the clothes that we own, and imagine how they will look on us once we lose the body fat that we intend on losing. If we know it will not fit us well after we make this transformation, then we must give them away now.

Likewise, we must go through our house and rid of all the unhealthy foods we know do not belong in our household. The more convenient it is to eat these foods, the more you will test your will power, and that is unnecessary. We want to create barriers and distance

147

between these fat-supporting foods and us. By doing so, we have to think and travel to the stores if we wish to buy these foods and drinks. Rid of all the biscuits, cakes, crisps, white bread, pastry, sweets, fizzy drinks and fruit juices in your fridge and cupboards. Make things simpler for yourself. Another strategy is to always pay good money for salad, vegetables, lean meats and nuts, and abstain from paying higher prices for foods that you know will make you gain weight. Furthermore, we can also make statements by investing in a personal trainer for many sessions. By making this commitment, we set the tone for the following weeks. We will be held accountable, and we must remain consistent.

Chapter 5: Psychology – Focus

Focus and Perception

"There is no truth. There is only perception." -
Gustave Flaubert

There is something to be learned in every single thing that we experience. It all comes down to how we choose to view what we encounter. Whether we conceive things positively or negatively will determine our direction, and, ultimately, our degree of success as it relates to our health and physical goals. What we focus on proliferates. We think around 60, 000 thoughts every day, most of which are repeated and often negative unless we work hard to condition ourselves. If we have more negative than positive thoughts, then it is only natural that we will end up attaching more emotions to negative thoughts. If they have any significance to us, then our thoughts lead to feelings, which lead to us taking actions (whether good or bad). Our physical shape depends on the emotions we choose to attach to our thoughts. This is why we must fully immerse ourselves in our positive thoughts, and take some form of action to support it as soon as possible.

We must give energy to things that empower us. If everyone looked into the sky, each individual would think of something distinct: "I wonder if that star still exists." "Why am I here?" "Should I marry him?" Should I divorce her?" "What is man's potential?" The same image can evoke any thought or feeling. Every single person conjures his or her subjective energy, depending on his or her perspective, and the influence of the ego. A perspective has infinite possibilities, yet we subjectively choose to think and feel a certain way. It is interesting how we can hear, see, feel, smell and taste the same things, yet interpret things differently depending on our mood at that moment, and how we link things together in our minds. We must change our associations and reactions if we are to take certain actions. For example, if we all tried to squeeze our bellies with our hands, then we are likely to think and feel a range of different things. Some might think, "this is not good enough," or "I am getting in better shape," or "I am surprised," or "I love having that extra layer of love!" If we want to get into even better shape, then we must accept ourselves as we are, but we must also feel some strong emotion and intensity to lose more fat. Consider your reactions to when you become aware of your body, and how you respond to yourself.

A relationship means to have a connection. We have relationships with people, but we also have relationships with food. A relationship depends on all the thoughts and feelings you have towards something. We all use food for something, but we must simplify our relationship with food as much as possible. Many people choose to use food as a way of changing their states. They feel exhausted or stressed or angry, and they eat for instant gratification. This is a recipe for disaster if we are looking to create amazing physical bodies. Others use the act of eating as a reason to stop doing work. It can be a form of procrastination depending on context. Everyone uses food for fuel, and to give us the nutrients we need to function properly. However, food and drinks affect us differently. High sugary foods and drinks can provide fuel for the short term, but over time, the frequent consumption of these foods actually make us feel more exhausted and lethargic. They may give us a boost for a couple of hours, but refined carbohydrates and sugary foods will not sustain our energy for long. This is why light meals that are highly alkaline can sustain our energy levels for days, weeks and months if we live by it. We must look at food and drink as simply a long-term energy source.

It is not what happens to us, but how we react to things that ascertain our physical shape. If we drop a cup, and it breaks, what are the possible causes? Nothing at all; maybe I should take it easy; I am an idiot; I must be tired; I was supposed to break that cup and so on. It all depends on what we say to ourselves. These effects can be impersonal (they place no real judgement on us), or they are personal (I dropped the cup because I always make mistakes, or I dropped the cup because I am clumsy). These personal effects include 'I' or 'I am,' and thus identity is attached to them, which can either be empowering or disempowering depending on the impositions suggested. We must be very careful with what we attach to our identities as it subconsciously communicates we that cannot change these things. Write a list of I ams that you believe about your health, eating habits and training habits.

It is fascinating how our perceptions to things can completely change over the course of our lives. What was once hated can one day be loved. What was once feared can one day be relished. What was once a weakness can one day become a strength. It is about not accepting that our current situation is permanent. Our perceptions also change depending on our priorities and stage in life. Fire can work with us or against us depending on how, when and where we use it. The same applies to everything. Peruse some of the things you once detested that you now appreciate or love doing. Examine some of the challenges you have overcome and why. These same strategies must be applied to your exercise and eating routines.

We believe what we see; we choose what we see; we see what we believe.

Our brains choose certain things to pay attention to every minute of every day depending on likes, desires, pleasures, relationships, tasks and so on. What we have plugged into our subconscious will dominate much of our day. There are so many things we do on a daily basis where our 'default' mode is left in control; we go on autopilot many times during the day especially when we do things that we are familiar with. This is why it is so important to condition our minds, and to be vigilant regarding how we think and feel throughout the day. If we focus on the insects in the grass, we will miss the birds in the sky. If we focus on the pain in the world, we will miss the bliss and giving that exists. Even though this is the luckiest time to ever be alive, focusing on the right things are harder now than at any other time in history due to the influx of technology and information bombarding us from everywhere. We must be able to keep our lives simple and clear, so that we can focus on things that will support our health-related goals.

The same applies intrinsically: if we focus on what is lacking in our lives, a six-pack or the benefits that derive from it, then our feelings will be negative. This will result in either inertia or unsupportive actions as we are acting out of desperation. When we chase something, it manages to run further away. Fortunately, if we think about the amazing things in our lives or the positive things that are happening around us (most of which we probably take for granted), then that will expand. Our thoughts, which are generated by both internal and external stimuli, affect our emotions, and our emotions determine our actions. These three processes circulate again and again, building momentum, consolidating the pattern and increasing the stakes day-by-day. Sometimes in life, we simply do not get things if we force them or want them too much. We must give everything we have to something worthwhile, but we must also keep things in perspective. What thoughts come to mind every day as it relates to your health and physical shape? What emotions do you experience as a result? How does it affect your actions? Does it make you go gym more or less? Does it make you pick healthier choices or not? Does it increase stress levels or make you more relaxed?

Mind your own business! We can achieve and keep the bodies we want if we are disciplined. Wish well for others, but do not become entrenched with what others are doing, unless we can, and should, support them or learn from them. When we focus on another person meticulously, we trip ourselves up in the process, especially if we are focusing on their problems or mishaps. We want to avoid drama, and people who are immature or who cannot put things into perspective. Great pain derives from being given things, and not having to work for them. Their willpower and appreciation diminishes. They have only known easy times, and so do not develop the kind of discipline, dedication and drive required to pursue greater accomplishments in every sense. The worst thing we can be is spoiled. Why? We have high expectations, but no real substance to acquire them on our own. This results in low self-esteem eventually and the development of a victim mentality when we start thinking about why things are not going our way. The spoilt victim is a recipe for disaster. This is why we must know our purpose, remain on our path and persevere. We must appreciate the small improvements we are making to our bodies, and reward ourselves accordingly to continue this momentum.

"Where attention goes, energy flows." Tony Robbins

Context Reframing

We must be able to change what things mean to us if we are to choose the answers that will serve us best. Everything in life has a positive outcome available. It all depends on how we experience it. We abide by the norms and rules within so many different contexts, which reduces the size of our inner and outer 'box' of possibilities. This, in turn, reduces our ability to think and behave outside of this 'box,' hence why people say things like, "I'm not creative." These people care too much about how others perceive them. If you feel as though you cannot make a mistake in front of someone, then it is clear that they do not have unconditional love for you. Anyone who does not have unconditional love for you is therefore untrustworthy, as you know they will never always be there for you as it is all about how you are within the rules of his or her own "box." How can they if they will leave, abandon, fire or boycott you if and when you make a mistake or if they deem that you are not good enough? Knowing whom to spend time with, and where to devote your energy is massively important for your health and fat-loss goals. The biggest reason why people cannot lose more fat or gain more muscle is predominantly because of their psychology, and our psychology is largely affected by our surroundings and lifestyles.

Reject negativity, and encourage positivity. Make your smaller achievements larger in your mind. It means you are one step closer to achieving your goals. It is all about building momentum every single day! This is how we maintain our inner energy and drive. Those who feel like they never achieve enough or do enough will have low energy because their daily thoughts and emotions are often unnecessarily harsh. Be proud and content with yourself if you know that you had a productive day. Forgive yourself when you are not at your best. Know that you may need to take a small step back and gather yourself. Surround yourself with positivity and optimism. If you do not know many positive, inspirational people, then listen to podcasts, interviews and so on from people who inspire and motivate you. Negativity is contagious, and so is positivity. Avoid jealousy and envy because they are really thoughts and feelings that support the notion that you are not successful enough or will never be where you want to be. Be happy for others because, firstly, that is the right thing to do, and, secondly, because you want others to send positive energy back to you when you also achieve that level of success and happiness. We attract what we put out, as taught in *The Secret*.

Be able to take something, anything, and present it to yourself more favourably and pleasantly. Ask yourself some of the following questions when something challenging occurs: "How can I grow from this?" "What can I learn from this?" "How can this benefit me?" "Why will this support me?" Only positive answers can derive from these encouragingly phrased questions. These questions ensure that we focus on possibility and remain centred. Simply choose positive emotions rather than disempowering ones. Understandably, it is impossible to not experience the full spectrum of emotions available to human beings. No one has that innate ability. There will be moments when we feel stressed, angry, sad, fearful, anxious and so on. The key is to only experience these emotions for brief moments. One of the main aspects of emotional intelligence is being able to quickly change our states. There is a difference between momentarily experiencing something negative and expanding the experience. The key to becoming enlightened is to make this negative experience last as minimally as possible. For instance, how long are you angry for when a driver disrespectfully drifts into your lane? For me, the displeasure literally lasts for a second, and then I detach myself from the situation, and remind myself that I cannot affect another person's actions, and I will not allow it to affect my experience, as they would win if I did. It is perilous to let another human being dictate our feelings especially for a sustained period of time. Instead, anticipate that we will encounter lunatics and awful drivers on our journeys; envision the best scenario, but be prepared for the worst. This is how we avoid disappointment, yet remain focused and driven to achieve the very best outcomes for our bodies and health: arriving safely at our destinations! We have control of it, and no one has the right to influence our thoughts and feelings.

How can we use our energy in more empowering and productive ways? Daily, weekly and monthly planning will keep us on track and centred. Make time for the things you love in order to increase your energy, so that you can deliver in all avenues passionately. I used to think I needed at least eight hours of sleep to functions well. Sometimes I would sleep for eight hours and still be tired! Now this may not be the case for some as a result of their poor eating and drinking habits, but I was still healthy, and yet unable to have that strong drive upon waking. That all changed when I had more exciting things to do! We know that we live captivating lives when we do not want to go to sleep (because we are excited about doing and creating things). The same applies for waking up. If we know that we have a lot of important and exciting things to do, then we really want to kick start our day. If we do not have this feeling, then we are not being as creative, driven and excited as we should and could be. What was once a weakness can become a strength. I have observed this in my own life within many different contexts: I once hated to exercise, and I use to avoid it at all costs; now I love to train, and do so daily with great pleasure and eagerness. Moreover, I once disliked reading, and was resistant when my mother encouraged me to read when I was a child; I now teach, read and learn for a living. I have never been happier. Do not fear what you initially do not like. It may one day turn out to be your greatest joy. These changes were only possible due to my desire to improve, and to not accept that I was incompetent at something. Move towards what you fear. Think about the exercises you least enjoy doing, and make them an integral part of your weekly workouts. Think about what healthy foods you know are healthy yet do not like tasting, and make it part of your weekly dish. You will learn to enjoy it, and thus become ever closer to getting the body you deserve.

Small Successes

We lose what we do not use. Muscles, skills, knowledge etc. are all lost over time unless we constantly reuse these influential assets. The same applies to our thoughts and emotions. If we do not show love, affection, intimacy, then we lose the ability to experience it fully and often. I like to use the muscle metaphor. If we gain a large amount of muscle, and then lose it, it is actually very easy to accumulate the same sized muscle again. It is called muscle memory. The same exists for what we feel. If we do not eat or train well, then we lose the ability to keep and build muscle. If we lose the ability to kiss, cuddle, laugh and so on, then we lose the ability to express and feel. We must constantly condition ourselves because we are creatures of habit. We must have the energy to sustain our habits. Every time we break a habit, we can become a little weaker with another supportive habit. This continuously goes up and down depending on our discipline. The more we keep our habits daily, the more often we deliver. Not doing seemingly innocuous things such as doing our beds in the morning, or brushing our teeth, or meditating, actually begins a cascade of broken promises to oneself. The next thing you know, you laid in bed instead of getting up to go gym. Subsequently, you fail to prioritise and complete the most important action of the day. Stick to your promises. If you consistently let yourself down, then you lose trust within yourself. Can you imagine what this does to your self-esteem? Our self-esteem is tied to our standards, and what kind of bodies we feel we deserve. The higher our self-esteem, the more hope we have of an even stronger and better body.

Success, in terms of our physical shape, is really an accumulation of small wins. Small things add up, which help us to accomplish the bigger things. If you ask a professional or master within a certain field, "what makes you outstanding?" do not expect an incredible mind-blowing response, as you are likely to be disappointed. Their response will leave you thinking, "Well, I can do those things as well, or most of them at least." The answer is yes you can, but most people do not because they are driven by a more fantastical dream: that outstanding achievers can do things that normal people cannot. Yes, people have varying degrees of talents and energy etc., but real success is not sexy at all. It is about grinding consistently. It is about showing up, and doing the small things ceaselessly regardless of how we feel.

159

Achievements create fleeting moments of happiness, but continual progression, in an area that we deem important, builds long-lasting happiness and strong self-esteem. What small things do you need to do on a daily basis, so that you can create your dream body and health? How can we implement these into our lives today?

The Mirror

Every time Susan went to look in the mirror, she was always instantly drawn to the parts of her body she did not like: her belly and love handles. Not only did she focus on these areas, but also she would always say to herself something along the lines of, "Why can't I lose weight here?" This question can only drive negative and hurtful responses: "Because I am lazy. Because I eat too many cakes. Because I never exercise. Because I'm weak." The mind tells your eyes to look at your problems (your belly and love handles), and your emotions are disempowering. No wonder why Susan never takes the necessary actions that can actually change her physical appearance. Next time you look in the mirror, focus only on the things that you like about yourself (or could like).

Interestingly, the more you focus on what you like about yourself (your eyes, lips, arms etc.), the more your weaknesses will improve because you naturally begin to make better choices as it relates to food choices, exercise, sleep etc. We gravitate toward what we want. For example, we often manage to bump into the people we like most at work or at a social gathering. Why? Because your energies aligned. Unfortunately, the same magnetic pull works if two people do not want to bump into each other. It is all about focusing on what you want, and deciding that this is the way it is going to be. The same applies to our habits. Focus on the brilliant or beneficial things you do every single day, and you will miraculously begin to implement even better habits in other areas. Some beneficial habits can be as simple as brushing our teeth, writing out our goals, showing someone how much we care about him or her or investing in something we know will support our fat-loss goals. What we focus on expands.

Questions

What we focus on is really determined by the quality of questions we ask ourselves. Our questions narrow the potential answers, so it is down to us to feed the mind positively phrased, powerful questions. If we do not like the answer, then we can change the question until we get the answers we want. We must start searching for the answers that support us. It does not matter if amazing answers do not come to us! We will condition our minds to constantly see the good in things. Our subconscious will soon take over, and we will find ourselves in more fortuitous circumstances. It is about training the mind to look for what it wants, and to reject barriers (some form of negativity). Either avoid the obstacle or walk through it. We cannot prevent negative thoughts all of the time, but we can control how we respond to these negative thoughts and questions. We must always question our negative thoughts or visualisations. What purpose do they serve? If you do not like the mind's projections, then we can correct them by diligently imagining and creating supportive notions and images.

Out of Sight, Out of Mind

Avoid seeing unhealthy foods where possible. Instead have healthy, constructive surroundings around you. Will power alone is not strong enough. We must ensure that our fridges and cabinets do not have unhealthy foods and drinks. It will only be a matter of time before we start justifying why we should eat some of them: "Oh it's not as bad as a massive cake. I can have a little." The more hesitation we put in our minds, the closer we are to succumbing. However, if our surroundings are healthy, organised and spacious, then we create the right kind of climate for a healthy lifestyle. Consider what your weekly shopping list contains. How many unhealthy foods could you supplant with healthier alternatives?

It is not just about what foods and drinks there are in the house. It is also about convenience. Ensure that there is easy access to healthy foods. If you have some unhealthy treats, then make them harder to access. For example, we should not have any treats already out on tables or worktops or in your main fridge. They are just constantly in our faces, and we move toward what we see more often. Additionally, ensure that we have to work for our treats. If you have any, then put them in your garage fridge or in the highest shelf of your cabinet. It should never be easy to grab them otherwise it will be just as easy to ruin our eating plans.

Similarly, be cautious with where you go out with friends and family. If you know the kind of areas they like to go, and what places are their favourites, then you can foresee what kind of temptations you might encounter. It is very important to know the psychology of your friends and family. What are they thinking? How do they try to present things to you in order to get you out? How do they excuse themselves for negative eating? Suggest areas where you know there are healthier alternatives. See if you can plan your socialising, and thus when you should have your cheat meal. If it is not part of your plan, and you know you could be tempted or coaxed into unhealthy eating and drinking, then avoid going out on that occasion. The more proactive we are, the more we will set ourselves up for success.

Our Beliefs

"You know you're in love when you can't fall asleep because reality is finally better than your dreams." – Dr. Seuss

What we believe will become our reality. If we believe in Islamic practices, then we are right. If we believe in Christianity, then we are right. If we believe in trust and honesty, then we are right. Whatever we believe to be the truth, the core of our existence, then we are right. Our internalisation is our truth. What do you believe about your potential, and how you can transform your body? We create our energy, and our effects on others. Our energy meshes with the universe's energy to affect others and us one way or another. If we believe it, so it shall be. Unfortunately, or fortunately, depending on how we are, people become rigid and stubborn in their thoughts and beliefs, which is harmful and perilous to the self: we limit what we can think, experience and share. We can only see one way, and even if we believe in a bigger cause, it is the ego that rears its ugly face whenever we undermine or belittle another's beliefs. The paradox is that we come to believe that we are always complete, yet whenever we stop learning and thinking, we metaphorically and spiritually die. We must be flexible in our beliefs, not necessarily docile and malleable, but capable of change. Anyone who stays the same no longer fits in today's ever-changing world. If we are inflexible, we will not progress. We must be like water. Do not work against what is natural. We all have a purpose, and an ability to profoundly affect others. We must decide what our ideal selves are, and make decisions based on these promising prototypes.

Physical muscles grow when they are pushed. The same exact principle applies to the mind. To break through we must become uncomfortable. Unfortunately, this is often when people stop, and they become helpless. It is because no character is being built when people do not break through. A weak character is a consequence of weak thoughts and weak standards. How do we know when we have broken through a metaphorical barrier? What is it that we always, or frequently, say to ourselves when we reach the peak of something difficult? "I can't swim another lap." "If I fail, I'll look stupid." "I've never been able to do it before." "I'm just not good at it." "This is enough for me." In these instances, the key words are obvious: "Can't," "stupid," "never," "not good" and so on. We must condition ourselves, so that when we reach these points, we automatically think something more inspiring and uplifting. The powerful words, "I am" must be followed with whatever positive phrases we want. Now that we are conscious of what we say when in these situations, we must apply a vibrant image of success in our minds, and affirm this chosen positive phrase over and over: "I am successful," "I am going to accomplish this," or even better, "I have already accomplished this." "I deserve this," "I always find a way." All we need to focus on is taking just one step at a time.

If we are struggling to tackle something challenging, then we should begin something even harder than what we already have as a barrier to our progression. Doing something even more dangerous or challenging brilliantly utilises the power of contrast. For example, if you thought running for four miles was hard, then wait until you sign yourself up for a marathon. If you thought a circuit class was challenging, then partake in a crazy cross-fit challenge. The initial task does not seem as daunting now. Even so, things always have a way of working out, if we can learn to have faith and work on what we value. Yes, we can dictate our life's journey, but to achieve this poetically, we must accept all that happens in our lives. Things can always have a beautiful spin to them (context reframing) if we so choose to give it one.

We all have thresholds for different things. Some thresholds are higher than others depending on our standards and priorities. The way to grow is to always place demands on these thresholds, always push slightly more each time until our previous threshold is no longer a barrier, and we can push further, experience newer, and, thus, be happier. Happiness is achieved by continuous growth in areas that we value. Happiness is not something we will attain one day, like a possession. Even if we think we will be permanently happy if we just lost a few pounds, and never had to train again, we would be wrong. Boredom, complacency and the subsequent negative thoughts will soon seep into our extra freedom unless we find new inspiring activities. We must constantly challenge and break barriers to sustain true contentment and inner peace. Think about your healthy eating barriers. How healthily do you eat, and how often do you really wish to have your cheat meal? This is your eating barrier. Peruse your exercise barriers. When is a gym workout enough? How many times must you train a week until you think, "that's enough for the week now." Challenge your barriers consistently.

Think about the physical journey we most often make: usually to a workplace, relative or friend. What we will notice is that our minds go on autopilot due to the familiarity of the scenery and routine. This creates comfort and relaxation, but will rarely ever fill us with new thoughts. However, when we explore an unfamiliar journey, our minds operate differently, often with randomness, and a whole range of extreme thoughts and emotions may pervade our mental fluency. Where there is chaos, there is a chance to create something new: a new belief. A challenge to customary thinking begins. This is how we live our own lives. We become complacent and unnecessarily comfortable. It is impossible to grow, progress and experience anew unless we travel down a different path (both physically and mentally). Think about the boring routines you have on a daily or weekly basis. How can we change them? How can we make things fresh, new and challenging? This is necessary if we want to change and shake some of our current key foundations. If we want a better body, especially if this requires a more radical transformation, then we must change our familiarities where possible. We must shift our identities if we are to shift our results.

Chapter 6: Psychology – Leadership

What is your Why?

In order to develop and keep the kind of body and health we deserve, we must have a big enough why. In order to lead ourselves, and others, we always must have a cultivating and enticing why. If we do not have powerful, intense emotions attached to a health-related goal, then we are unlikely to persevere when things are not going as planned or if unexpected things get in the way. If your why is massive and robust, then you will find a way! We need to inspire ourselves. So what is your why? Why do you want to lose fat, and become a healthier person? Is it so that you can live longer, and enjoy more special moments with loved ones? Is it so that you can be more active now and later in life, so that your activities will not be as compromised? Is it so that you will look better and stronger in order to attract a better quality partner? Is it so that you can be an even better role model for your children? Is it to overcome an illness? We must revisit this why every single time we are working toward its attainment. We must use this why even after we have achieved the goal because once it is achieved, we can always raise the bar higher. It does not have to stop there. If we are not getting better, we are getting worse.

Leadership

"A leader is best when people barely know he exists...when his work is done, his aim fulfilled, they will all say: We did it ourselves." – Lao-Tzu

Leadership is one of the most important aspects of developing an incredible body. Leadership is all about being able to influence ourselves, and then being able to influence others. We need to know how to lead ourselves, and how to influence others, so that they support our healthy lifestyles. If the leader is not at work, then the employee will still arrive early, put in a shift, behave professionally and they will feel empowered to do their job brilliantly. If the leader is not with their friends, then his or her friends will still speak highly of the leader when the leader is not around; they have the leader's back, and will defend the leader if another person does not speak well of him or her. If the leader is not with his or her child, then the child will do the right thing, and will avoid rebelling and doing scandalous things because the child values himself or herself, and wants to represent the family well. Now think about what leadership does to you. The better the leader, the more disciplined, responsible and focused the person must be. These are probably the three most important things we need if we are to have an amazing body: we must be consistent and embed many healthy routines every single day to strengthen our resolve; we must be accountable for the decisions we make, and for the results we generate; we must be so focused that we begin to create opportunities that we never even considered.

Leaders (not managers) and winners always find a way to get the job done! So how does the brain work when tackling something challenging or arduous, such as staying on the right eating schedule or getting ready for a tough workout when you are already tired? We tend to go through the same sort of cycle when doing things that are taxing and tough: we usually start things well (due to our enthusiasm, and the novelty of what is being done), and then we reach a moment where it suddenly becomes really challenging (mostly because something dawns on us that we did not foresee, or something was harder than we thought it would be); during this moment, we start to question the activity, and ourselves, much more: "I don't know if I have enough time to complete the whole workout today," or "I have been eating well for a few days now, and I really want to just let loose. Maybe I am just not cut out for this lifestyle." The interesting thing is that if we somehow manage to be resilient in these moments (by calming ourselves down; mustering enough mental and physical energy to continue and so on), then we will notice that the 'hardest part' (especially nearer the end of the hardest part) suddenly becomes a lot easier, and we end up doing better than we thought.

"People who are truly strong lift others up. People who are truly powerful bring others together." – Michelle Obama

Responsibility

"You cannot escape the responsibility of tomorrow by evading it today."
– Abraham Lincoln

People who have managed to sustain a sexy and strong body for many years always take responsibility whether things are going well or badly in their personal and professional lives, or whether they are winning or losing. Leaders never claim to be the helpless victim. They never come up with weak excuses by pointing the finger at others. They know that if they ruined their eating plans or evaded going to the gym for too long, then it was their own fault. Leaders always have options and choices because they are versatile, and they manage to create a new way if their main plans are not going as expected. The person who refuses to take responsibility will suffer from the 'victim syndrome.' We are powerful human beings who always manage to manifest the energy within ourselves to step up whether we feel like it or not. We must believe that we are responsible for our actions.

Once we take responsibility for our actions, routines and reactions, then we begin to make personal improvements. Leaders know that they always have a choice. We choose where we direct our energy and focus. When we take responsibility, we feel empowered and in control. The externals should never dictate our intrinsic beliefs, and the way we should live our lives. External things or people are never to blame for our current health and physical situations as we must be strong enough to dictate our own journeys. When we blame externals, we communicate that we are not in charge. This is a destructive and pessimistic viewpoint. Resist the decadent urge to blame society, politics, our partners, siblings or friends. This is taking the easy way out. Nothing worth living for is easy. We must be intrinsically impregnable, and always look inward rather than outward if something does not go our way.

Decision-Making

"Inability to make decisions is one of the principle reasons executives fail. Deficiency in decision-making ranks much higher than lack of specific knowledge or technical know-how as an indicator of leadership failure." – John C. Maxwell

The more quickly we follow our intuition when deciding upon something, the more efficiently and clearly our brains will operate. The more we hesitate, the more uncertain we become in other areas. The more we question something, the weaker it becomes. If we want to develop this ability, then, as with everything, we must start small. When making small-scale decisions, such as what to eat today, or what to wear, we must condition ourselves to make the decision immediately. People overthink and spend way too much time contemplating things that are insignificant. We also teach the brain to never be assertive and decisive whenever we do this. They psych themselves out. They prevent any opportunity to experience flow, which is all about minimising our conscious mind, and allowing our unconscious qualities and mechanics to come out magnificently.

Intuition should always surmount contemplation. Our intuition is our gut feeling, which involves our subconscious perceptions. Follow this every single time. A general rule of thumb is to make up our minds within ten seconds, regardless of how monumental the decision. Leaders are decisive, and we want to lead our lives with confidence. We might make fewer mistakes if we always question what we are doing (such as question why we are eating healthily all the time, or why we must go gym every couple of days), but we will miss out on the best opportunities if we have to always double check and question things. Yes, it can be beneficial to write down the pros and cons of our options, but people are capable of making quality decisions rapidly. It just takes practice and conditioning. Here are some things to practice before embarking on bigger decisions: what do you want to eat for breakfast tomorrow? Decide in five seconds. How much fat do you want to lose by December? Decide in five seconds. What outfit do you want to wear for your next night out? Decide in five seconds. Power comes from being certain and decisive. Take control now.

Prioritise

"The key is not to prioritize what's on your schedule, but to schedule your priorities." –
Stephen Covey

The main reason why people do not develop the kind of body they desire is because it is not a priority for them. It must become a must for us. Every day consists of just twenty-four hours, and we can only do so much within that time. We only have time for our main priorities, and it is up to us to determine what those are. We must take our fat-loss goals seriously enough to put it alongside some of our biggest concerns. Whilst it is important to build upon our successes, we should always have one thing that takes precedence, for a certain period of time, because this is how we master a skill. Our priorities require immersion and great focus. We must also be realistic. Alternate when to prioritise different things. Know when to put muscle development first; know when to put healthy eating first; know when to put your finances first. Also, know what to always keep as a secondary focus point: something that is beneficial, but should never become a priority. Our hobbies and interests are secondary. Our family, health and finances are primary-focus areas. It can be beneficial to write out a schedule for the year, knowing when to prioritise different things depending on key events and times of the year. We might also want to plan how our training and eating plans might change.

Do what is important first, and not what is urgent. If urgent things pop up frequently, then we are probably being too reactive and not proactive enough. We must be able to anticipate what issues might come up in different areas, and have time and systems set up to deal with its apparition. Things that are important are usually long-term activities that are related to our biggest goals. Things that are urgent and that do not hold great significance are short-term tasks that often require our present moments for brief periods of time. Aim not to give substantial time to what is urgent. There is a massive difference between what is important and what is urgent. We can greatly reduce what is urgent by being more proactive. If many urgent things show up frequently, then it will add to our stress levels, and we know by now that stress induces unhealthy choices and reactions: overeating, smoking, drinking, arguments, tension, negativity and so on.

How can we become more proactive? When we think about something, say our daily eating schedule, consider the next two or even five steps needed; think of it like playing a chess match. Anticipate any issues that may pop up within our relationships or business that might affect our food choices, or when we will or will not eat, and what we can put in place just in case. Maybe it is to have our meals preplanned and made already. Maybe it is to have a coffee for a certain time when you know you will be too busy to eat. It is very easy to be distracted by what is urgent, but if we have a schedule, then we can still focus a lot of our time on the things that are important, so that urgent matters never drastically ruin our priorities. Additionally, we must know when we are most productive during the day (when we have most mental energy), whether in the morning, during the day or at night, and we must consistently dedicate this time to what is important. If we give our best to things that are only urgent, then it will take us much longer to accomplish our long-term goals.

People get stressed because of an accumulation of things (often urgent things). When we allow ourselves to be overwhelmed, we end up not doing anything at all, and we just worry and fret instead. This is when the mind wanders, and this is when we then procrastinate. What is the worst part? Many people are so busy doing things that they do not want to do, that they spend little time on things that mean a lot to them. They have not taken care of themselves first, and are putting other people's wants above their own, which indicates a lack of self-esteem and control in one's life. This results in long-term insufficient fulfillment, and thus overeating for example. However, some people use it as an excuse not to do more meaningful things because of some form of fear. Others get stressed and indignant as a result of never completing what they really want, and thus never experience what Maslow calls self-actualisation. We simply cannot experience the blissful state of self-actualisation (and its naturally enriching healthy behaviours) if we have not fulfilled the preceding human needs first...

Firstly, let us focus on the physiological needs. Yes, we all understand that we need to stay warm, sheltered, fed, rested and so on. Unfortunately, business-oriented and stressed individuals often neglect this basic stage because they are so obsessed with the later stages (significance in particular). Regrettably, this mentality is unsustainable in the long-term. We need to develop and embed regular patterns for these basic needs that are often taken for granted, so that we do not have to think about them, and thus detract focus from more meaningful things. We must have regular sleeping patterns; we must have specific eating schedules, and preferably certain, simple, repetitive meals in place (unless others cook for us) and so on.

Secondly, we all need to feel safe. Whilst this stage can refer to physical safety (and this is true), we must appropriately interpret this stage as referring to our mindset also. Do you feel in control of your life? Do you feel stable? Do you feel like you are certain about what your future will be like? Once we feel physically and mentally safe, we can begin to take control of our existence, and really instill quality supportive healthy strategies. Once we feel mentally and physically safe, we can then look outward. Consider your limiting beliefs and where they developed. We will want to address them at this stage healthily if we are to progress onto the other stages more effectively and robustly.

Thirdly, we all have the desire to feel loved or at least connected to others. Our inner primitive brain (that we all have biologically) will never allow us to be self-actualised unless we feel part of a troop. Many people are too nice, and they feel as though everyone in society should be part of their troop. This is ignorantly perilous. There are only a few people who should form part of our troop (our closest family members and friends). These are the only people who we should want to impress because these are the people who realistically give us, or should give us, unconditional love. However, we should care much less about what others think about us. Our loved ones support us, motivate us, and, therefore, enable us to develop the desire to excel without fear. Consider the people you would trust with all your money. Consider the people with whom you would risk your life for. These are the people who are part of your inner circle. Choosing unwisely can lead to a lot of pain, trauma and thus psychological problems that will negatively affect our health and body shape.

Fourthly, we have esteem needs. Once we feel appreciated and loved, then we are able to thrive and feel significant. This need is all about flourishing. We have the foundations in place: we feel physically and mentally strong and safe. We know that we are loved no matter what, that people are there to catch us if we fall, and so we have the inner strength to really go for what we want. We look to become the masters in our given fields at this point. We want to prove ourselves to the world. We want to feel significant. We turn our attention to what completes, inspires and drives us on our journey to freedom. We become consumed with business, financial matters and with getting further ahead. This is sometimes when many people either automate many healthy strategies, so that they can maintain a healthy and strong body whilst they pursue wealth and power, or this is when people sideline their health and body shapes in order to excel financially. This choice is incredibly important because it is like quicksand. If we lose control of our physical shape, then matters will worsen because we become even more obsessed with providing for our families financially or wanting to show off our qualities to others and ourselves.

Fifthly, we have finally arrived. This is the pinnacle. This is where we should all want to be. We now shift from being obsessed and preoccupied with ourselves to now giving to others and not just those within our troops. Firstly, we wish to help and love those in our inner circles. We then desire to positively affect as many people as we can because we empathise with others' pains and misfortunes. This can be in the form of giving products and services for free, or being philanthropic, or supporting others who have great altruistic intentions. Not everyone makes it to this stage, but this is the stage that contains the most peace and satisfaction. This is the stage where we feel as though it is not about us anymore. We have accumulated all the toys and material goods we always wanted. This is where we get bored of all our material luxuries, and we look for greater meaning and depth in our later years.

Let us perceive Maslow's hierarchy of needs as a kind of force field around us. It is really all about the quality and quantity of energy we have and share. When we are working on our basic needs (physiological and safety), our energies, our bubbles if you will, are only within us. We are unstable, insecure, vulnerable, and thus we cannot support anyone or anything else. When we move onto our psychological needs (the love and esteem areas) our 'bubbles' become bigger, and our energies shift to our friends, family and those who benefit in terms of clients, colleagues and employees. At the self-fulfillment stage, we are so strong and successful that we now give for the sake of giving, and our bubble is unlimited. We no longer focus on ourselves, and our main drive is to change communities, countries or maybe even the world. Think about your journey: what has it been like so far? How is this affecting your weight and health? What can you do to improve the quality of your life stage, and thus your physical shape? Things are more connected than we can ever imagine.

Honesty

"Love your Enemies, for they tell you your Faults." - Benjamin Franklin

Honesty is not only imperative when communicating with people, but even more of a necessity when communicating with ourselves. Mental and physical health (and its consequential fat-loss capabilities) is about the brutally honest communication between the different areas within our brains: our ids need to be fulfilled (the need for immediate protection and pleasure), and our superegos (strong, core beliefs and true identity) need expression also. Our egos are where these two areas meet, and a decision must be made. The more honest these three areas are with each other, the more smoothly they will exchange, which will enable mental and emotional balance. This will give us the strength required to make the best choices more often. If the id always wins, then we suffer long term; if the superego always wins, then we always feel like things are too strict and rigid. If you know yourself well enough (your beliefs, how you react, your mood, what is on your mind etc.), then you will be in a place to make better decisions for your health and body.

In many ways, the people who have hurt us the most are the people we owe the most. Regardless of how much pain or displeasure they may have caused, they have revealed the weaknesses within us. We all have weaknesses. Fortunately, the more we self-reflect, and make necessary changes, the less likely others will need to say and do to humble us into making the necessary changes. Maybe the man did not need to go through that divorce, if he simply took the time to understand his partner better and was attentive to his partner's needs. Maybe the woman did not need to have that car accident if she just listened to her friends who told her that she drives recklessly and impatiently. Maybe if the man listened more to others, then he would not attract so many painful and troublesome occurrences. It is very important to spot the small things that foreshow the more ominous things that will loom in the future unless we make the changes required. Be vigilant, reflective and therefore proactive. Make the appropriate changes now rather than simply denying or justifying its inevitability.

Inner Workings

"Control of consciousness determines the quality of life."
- Mihaly Csikszentmihalyi

Whenever our inner voice says something disconcerting or disparaging, ask it a question: "How does this help me?" And if it does not, which is usually the case, then simply acknowledge the thought, but appease it by providing evidence of times when things went well in similar situations, or remind it that you have certain skills to help in these situations. Strong, concrete evidence and affirmations will calm this fearful voice. For example, if you are about to partake in a really challenging workout, and something in your mind says, "You are not feeling your best. Are you sure you really want to train today? You know it is going to be really hard." What is this purpose of these interrogatives and derogative statements? Reply with something inspirational and supportive, "I am experienced and strong enough to always find a way to finish the workout," or "I am doing the best with what I have at this moment in time, and that is enough for me." Proactively prepare for any negative thoughts to occur before beginning an activity especially one that is significant. Know that you will hear these negative statements and questions before planning a healthy meal or before going to the gym. Remember that it all changes during the process; we begin to 'open up,' and enjoy eating the healthy meal or training hard at the gym. Understand that it is all part of the process. We just need to show up every single time.

Leaders know that a negative voice will appear at some point during the process, and so they prepare themselves to deal with this. Being able to dictate and control your physical body and health largely depends on your mentality. If we are to sustain an amazing body, we will need to experience a variety of different training and eating programs over decades. We therefore need to adapt well to new information and activities. Leaders have strong meta-cognition: they know how they learn best, and what procedures to follow. They look to find similarities between activities, so that they can transfer existing skills and knowledge to new situations. Unfortunately, many people are fearful when first learning something or doing something new because they are uncomfortable with change. They may fear what others will say and think, or feel inadequate and out of their depth due to past conditioning or experiences. They may think things like, "This will take me a long time to develop," "I don't know about this," "What if I fail?" "What's hard about this?" and so forth. These punitive declarative and interrogative statements already implant the notion that this person is excessively challenged and incapable of achieving in this activity now or later. In contrast, the successful, natural person will approach new experiences and challenges more positively, knowing they will not do brilliantly first time around, and so they are less tense during unfamiliar situations. They may think things like, "How can I do this really well?" "I have all these strengths in other areas, which is why I will be great at this also," "I am intelligent, so will automatically be able to surmount this," or "I always manage to find a way, so I will be fine," and so on.

Long-Term Thinking

"Long-term, we must begin to build our internal strengths. It isn't just skills like computer technology. It's the old fashioned basics of self-reliance, self-motivation, self-reinforcement, self-discipline, self-command." – Steven Pressfield

The ability to continuously think long-term will ascertain your level of success physically. Most people are either short-term thinkers generally or long-term thinkers generally. If I asked you to describe or draw a picture of a short-term thinker, and write down what you think their average week is like, then that would it be like? It would be extremely different if I asked you to describe or draw a long-term thinker. We must develop the mentality that we think long-term in all matters in order to establish congruency and to keep us consistent. For example, we must think long-term when it comes to our health, our physical shape, our careers, an investment, a partner, a place to live, how many children we want and so on. Short-term thinkers are dabblers: they will attempt something with the mentality that they need quick gains or must see big transformations immediately. As they will unlikely see these advancements quickly, then they will give up prematurely. They will make decisions that they will later regret. Distinctly, long-term thinkers have conditioned themselves to be patient and thus have better timing. They do not jump into a relationship with the first person they get along with; they do not start a diet really intensely, and give up two weeks later; they do not attempt to start a business, and give up at the first hurdle. Long-term thinkers are proactive. Because they plan ahead so well, they are aware of many mental and physical obstacles that await them.

Short-term thinkers tend to achieve the least in life. They do not put their rubbish away (because that takes effort); they do not start drawing that artwork because it takes too long (because it takes mental effort); they do not get out of bed early enough upon waking, even though they want to set up their own business (because that means no late-night fun). They require, and rely on, luck to actually achieve anything. Playing the lottery and betting is for the short-term thinker. It is the mental game of the working, lower and middle class because it is the easy way to acquire big money. They feel like the world owes them. It seldom works.

What are long-term thinkers like when it comes to six-pack thinking? Expectedly, long-term thinkers know how to motivate themselves: they know that if you quit an important activity today, then you can easily quit again in the near future. They know that if they eat a cake today, when it was not scheduled in the diary, then they know they are more likely to be impulsive on another occasion (as we experience many of the same thoughts and feelings every single day). They lose trust in themselves. If the majority of people experience similar thoughts and emotions every day, then they can anticipate when they are more likely to be weaker and give in to externals such as junk food and sugary drinks. Short-term thinkers will react to this thinking, "That is a bit harsh. It is only one cake! I mean is it really necessary to be like that?" The answer is yes. If you can be so easily swayed, by yourself or others, then you have no chance of making this a long-term transformation. We must set higher standards, and we must understand why it is so important to never give in. Keep the foundations strong.

Will my social life be affected? Yes, to an extent. Is it worth it? Well that is up to you. It all depends on how well you know yourself. If you are someone who will go out to a restaurant unsure of what you will have to eat, then you are in trouble. If you go out to a party, and you do not know if you will be drinking alcohol or not, then you are in trouble. If you are docile and someone who can get swayed by friends, peers or strangers when you go out for dinner or drinks, then you must plan these events as being a cheat meal, and also go out less frequently. However, if you know that you will order something healthy when out with friends and family, then by all means go out to dinner and have a great time. The same applies to all social occasions. Know how your brain works. Know if externals can change your internals, and make the choices based on your priorities.

Take a moment to consider your current thinking and emotional tendencies. What long-term routines and strategies do you currently incorporate as it relates to your fat-loss and muscle development goals? What other long-term beliefs and routines can you implement to improve the quality of your health and body? When can these be embedded into your daily or weekly schedule? How might they positively or negatively affect your current daily and weekly activities? Take a moment to evaluate what is possible, and which activities should take precedence.

Emotional Intelligence

"What really matters for success, character, happiness and life long achievements is a definite set of emotional skills – your EQ — not just purely cognitive abilities that are measured by conventional IQ tests." - Daniel Goleman

Emotional intelligence is the main skill required in the pursuit of an attractive, strong and healthy body. There is no doubt about it. Emotional intelligence is incredibly broad, yet we will condense it for the purposes of this book. Firstly, what is emotional intelligence? It is the ability to notice and control our emotions; it is the ability to create and sustain great relationships due to one's empathy and quality social skills. In terms of our own emotions, it is about knowing why we feel a certain way, how we operate, how we learn, what is important to us, and how to motivate ourselves. We must learn to continuously develop this trait if we are to maximise our potential. Secondly, we now need to peruse how we are with our emotions. I am about to present you with different scenarios, and I want you to score yourself out of ten (one being unaffected, and ten being extremely emotional).

1) How would you feel if a reckless, insensitive driver cuts you off on the road? Decide in ten seconds, and provide a score.

2) How would you feel if a customer rejects you? Decide in ten seconds, and provide a score.
3) How would you feel if you hear that a coworker was badmouthing you? Decide in ten seconds, and provide a score.
4) How would you feel if a partner or family member was angry with you, and you knew that you were in the right? Decide in ten seconds, and provide a score.
5) How would you feel if you lost thousands of pounds in an investment? Decide in ten seconds, and provide a score.

If you scored three or lower for all questions, then you can clearly control your emotions. Now let us explore some different scenarios, as it relates to the health and fitness world, but this time I hope that you experience stronger emotional responses rather than indifference. Be totally honest, and score yourself out of ten (one being unaffected, and ten being extremely emotional).

1) How would you feel if you miss a workout? Decide in ten seconds, and provide a score.
2) How would you feel if you ruined your healthy-eating program, and it was not meant to be a cheat meal? Decide in ten seconds, and provide a score.
3) How would you feel if you trained even harder than expected? Decide in ten seconds, and provide a score.
4) How would you feel if you fitted into a certain-sized outfit that you always wanted to wear? Decide in ten seconds, and provide a score.

5) How would you feel if you lost a couple pounds this week in bodyfat? Decide in ten seconds, and provide a score.

Hopefully you scored seven or above for those questions. Emotional intelligence is about controlling our negative thoughts and emotions, yet being able to express positive, joyous thoughts and emotions to the fullest. The happier and more optimistic we are, the more weight we can shift. The more negative and pessimistic we are, the harder it is to lose fat because we have all kinds of energies and stresses now working against us.

High Self-Esteem

"You yourself, as much as anybody in the entire universe, deserve your love and affection" – Buddha

There are certain societal and cultural ideologies that simply limit our quality of life. When was it conceited or wrong to love yourself? Now arrogance and rudeness are not the most pleasant or attractive qualities to possess, but that does not mean that we should not appreciate who we are. We must love ourselves completely; we must believe in our potential to do more and become more; we must go for what we want, and love ourselves even if we do not achieve as much as we want. Know that you deserve everything you want. Unfortunately, many people have accepted low energy; they have accepted mediocrity in every aspect of life. This is incredibly sad. You can still be a good person, and yet have a thriving business. You can still be a humble person, and have the most gorgeous six-pack. You can still be a respectful person, and still be absolutely obsessed with chasing your dreams.

One of the reasons why people do not have the kind of body they want is because they think that others will disapprove of the changes they have made both mentally and physically. This is not about what others will think about you; this is about what you think of yourself. Another reason why people do not have the kind of body they want is because they operate at the same emotional frequency as the average person who is just content with being average. You are not average if you have an amazing body. Life and society will generally reward you more for being more attractive and powerful. A third reason why people do not have a great body is because they have accepted their limiting beliefs about what they can achieve. I can use every excuse out there as to why I should not have a ripped, attractive body, but excuses are for the weak. I was an obese teenager. Everyone within my immediate family, and most of my relatives, are overweight. I have other priorities, and a business to run. It is very easy to think, "It is only a matter of time before I return to being overweight," or "My family is this way, and that is the way I am meant to also be," or "I am incredibly hard working, and I just do not have the time to do everything I want for my body." Excuses are everywhere, but leaders are not. Know what you want, and refuse to let limitations stop you.

Go Big

"The future belongs to those who believe in the beauty of their dreams."
- *Eleanor Roosevelt.*

Why settle for just having a decent body? It does not matter whether you are already in good shape or if you have one hundred pounds you wish to shed, either way we must set big goals for our health and physical shape. Everyone's body is different. It is up to us, alongside any other professional help, to understand how our bodies react to different 'diets' and training methods. This is all about trial and error because there is so much content out there, and much of it is contradictory. Once we learn what works for us, then we need a bespoke eating and training schedule that we must automate. We must be consistent and disciplined. Think about the body you want, and double its quality and look. Most people do not know what they are capable of achieving. If we remain focused, and seek help along the way, then nothing can stop us. We want to inspire, challenge and give ourselves every opportunity to create the life we deserve.

In order to drastically change our lives, depending on our current physical appearance and health, then we must literally become a new person. Our personality is comprised of our beliefs, our thoughts, our emotions and our behaviours. If we need to change something really meaningful to us, such as our bodies, then we must rewire our identity and our personality. It sounds daunting, but it is necessary if we wish to cultivate greatness. If we think similar thoughts every day, and we experience similar emotions every day, and we do similar things every day, then these all culminate to determine who we are. We must question our thoughts. You may benefit from simply siting in silence and writing down the thoughts that come to mind. Afterwards, you can highlight the positive things that came to mind along with the negative things in another colour. You will learn a great deal about yourself from this very awkward experience. We must rewrite the script, so that we think positively and optimistically where possible. Once we change our thoughts, we can then focus on our emotions. What are we feeling? Write these down. Highlight as before. Write out what emotions you could supplant and why. Perusing our thoughts, emotions and behaviours will enable you to literally change your personality. If we do not wish to change our personalities, then that is fine, but understand that you will not be able to achieve massive changes in your life by remaining as you are now. The choice is yours.

Learn from Mistakes

"We are products of our past, but we don't have to be prisoners of it."
- Rick Warren

I have made so many dietary and exercising mistakes over decades. I have learned so much in terms of exercise technique, effects on metabolism, what certain foods contain and will do to our bodies, and how to structure my physical aspirations around other priorities. Most of the strategies I employ are now automated; I do not have to put in any mental or emotional work to complete the activities whether it is eating certain meals or training certain times or adhering to my morning and bedtime routines. It is so easy for me now, but many routines are conspicuously tough initially. You are on your individual path. The more actions you take, the more mistakes you will make, and the more quickly you will learn. There is no one size fits all when it comes to our health and physical shape, as there are too many variables. It is important to learn from others' mistakes, but sometimes from our own as well. This is unavoidable. The main thing is to constantly learn and challenge yourself.

If something is not going well in terms of your eating habits or training, then change it as soon as you can. The definition of insanity is doing the same thing over and over again, and expecting a different result. If we know that there is an unsupportive habit that we must change, then we have to attack it from different angles, and seek support if necessary. Think about what happens to our psychology if we know that we keep making the same mistakes that jeopardise our physical goals and health. Think about what it does to our self-esteem. Think about what it does to our belief in ourselves. Identify the problems, and do whatever necessary to change them. You might want to focus on changing one negative habit per week, as we do not want to overload ourselves. Write down a list of unhelpful things that you do. Do you tend to overeat or eat unhealthily when you get back from work? Do you keep saying that you will train after work, but never do because you are exhausted after work? Do you keep saying that you will get a personal trainer, but never go ahead with it? Do you keep saying that you want to wake up earlier and meditate or exercise before you begin your active day? Evaluate and order these habits in terms of how much you think they hinder your fat-loss endeavours. Write a weekly list of the one thing you will change each week. Reward yourself every week that you have changed that habit.

Master Strengths; Delegate Weaknesses

"A person's strength was always his weakness,
and vice versa."
- Viet Thanh Nguyen

Everyone has some strengths, as it relates to one's health and physical attributes. Maybe you have fast twitch muscles. Maybe you have long legs. Maybe you are very flexible. Maybe you have great endurance. Maybe you are very disciplined. Maybe you have a strong psychology. Maybe you are studious, and seek support and knowledge from others. Take a moment to write down the physical and mental aptitudes you possess. How can you amplify these strengths? How can you use them to your advantage? This will build momentum, and make you enjoy the activities that make you feel confident.

As it relates to our weaknesses, we have two options. Firstly, we can attack these weaknesses ourselves in order to improve them. This can be in the form of studying, researching, learning, self-reflecting, embedding habits ourselves such as changing our shopping lists or training more independently and so on. Secondly, we can look to delegate or seek support from professionals. If we dislike cooking for ourselves, then have someone cook for you. If we want to change our eating program, then we can hire a nutritionist. If we do not have the discipline to train on our own, then we can train with friends or get a personal trainer. We must know when to ask for assistance. It does not matter how strong the ship is, if there are enough holes in the ship, then it will sink.

Chapter 7 – Energy

Health

"I believe that the greatest gift you can give your family and the world is a healthy you." – Joyce Meyer

Much of the happiness and health we experience comes down to our relationship with food. The more energy we have, the more open we are to experiencing positive, upbeat thoughts and feelings. It does not matter how intelligent we are, if we are fueling our bodies and brains with garbage, then we are crippling our ability to consistently perform at our best. Our eating lifestyle has a profound effect upon our serotonin levels and our general wellbeing. We are all humans, and so we all experience similar emotions. Just because I am a positive and enlightened being, does not mean that I never experience a negative thought or emotion; the only difference is how this negative fabrication affects me. It never immobilises me. In fact, whenever experienced, it spurs me on and motivates me. A negative moment is just that: a moment. This massively relates to our emotional intelligence: the more quickly we are able to change and manipulate our states, the easier it is to take control of our experiences, and therefore do the best things more often. Refuse to allow a detrimental thought or emotion to affect you for a long period of time. We should never entertain something that has no value to us. On a different note, even the most positive and energetic person will experience lethargy. Whenever the mind or body is exhausted, then it is almost impossible to feel empowered, positive and inspired. This is why eating properly is crucial for daily mental and physical optimisation. Consider your eating plan, and evaluate whether you have a balance diet of essential macronutrients and micronutrients.

How do we know if we are living prosperously? Is it based upon the minimal moments of ecstasy experienced when we attain something, like a promotion, the birth of our children, fleeting intimate experiences with a partner? Is this how we evaluate success? Or do we attain happiness by having what others want and value such as mansions, flashy cars, a trophy wife or husband? True happiness is about maintaining energy and positivity on a daily basis for long periods such as months and years. It is what we feel during the most familiar processes of our daily lives. I call it our base mood or default emotion. We can partly 'set' our default emotion (to be happy, peaceful or joyous) by consuming high-quality, healthy foods and drinks. The immediate experience determines if we feel happy, and to win the ultimate game of life, we must be able to experience satisfaction and happiness every day for as long as possible. This can only be achieved through the energy that we have on a daily basis as energy changes our thoughts, our emotions and subsequently our actions. Therefore, what we eat and drink largely determines our personalities.

Eating well and healthily is a way of cultivating success. One of the most important moments in my life was when

I began to really eat well (even though I thought I had been eating well previously) and take care of my body to the maximum (by listening to how it feels). Thankfully, I decided to consume primarily earth-grown foods and drinks. Joyfully, I noticed that I had a greater desire to learn things. I noticed that I became even more loving and giving to others. I became less anxious or stressed out with many diverse things. Furthermore, I not only developed the discipline required to remain focused on what truly matters in life (family, friends, giving, health and wealth), but I was giving my mind and body what it needs to feel lighter, and to think more clearly. My memory improved, and so has my self-esteem.

Really, eating well and exercising well require the same belief. It is all about focusing on our behaviours just one day at a time. Understandably, it is important to know how we want to eat and exercise in the long term, but the only way to stay on track is to focus on the next step. It is important to set huge long-term goals, but we must live within the present moment because that is all we ever have. If we go for a run, and we are becoming increasingly exhausted, then all we need to do is focus on moving our legs for the very next step. If we are overly concerned with the entire run, then we may psyche ourselves out. Similarly, if we are looking at that cake, then all we need to do is focus on our very next move: bypass the cake, and opt for the salad. Forget thinking about healthy eating for the rest of the day or the entire week; just avoid that moment of potential weakness, and get through it without any damage! Interestingly, our desire for that cake will subside quite quickly once we move on. Only think about getting through that brief moment of impulsivity. It never lasts long. Do not allow your brain to trick you!

Exercise consistently, both moderately and intensely, to increase your energy levels. Stretch and move your body every day. Just focus on turning up at the gym. It is half the battle. Aim to beat existing physical, and mental, aptitudes by setting bigger goals and reflecting over your performances. What has allowed you to lift heavier? What has enabled you to run for longer? What has enabled you to rest less in between sets? However, never let exercise weaken the mind: overtraining can hinder any possible physical and/or mental gains. It can also lead to fatigue and uncontrollable overeating. Listen to your body: if it is excessively sore, then rest. Otherwise you will stress the mind, as the mind will have to work harder to keep you on track.

Incidentally, those who view themselves as doing better than they actually did in an activity are more likely to continue partaking in that same activity. We gravitate to what we are good at. That is just natural. In contrast, those who evaluate themselves realistically do not exhibit the same amount of enthusiasm to continue with their efforts. Therefore, it is better to be optimistic than realistic especially when embarking on acquiring new skills. Accentuate your strengths to yourself, and this will give you the boost to persist in an activity, such as exercising, so that you can develop the resilience needed to deal with adversity unwaveringly. See yourself performing better than you actually did. Even if you know it is an exaggeration, it is still worthwhile because you manage to manipulate yourself masterfully. You begin to envision greater success and positive performances, which spurs more positive thinking, emotions and further actions. It maintains the belief that you can do even better, and that your qualities are limitless. Actions and reflection will inevitably lead to success.

Alkaline

"NO disease, including cancer, can exist in an alkaline environment."
– Dr. Otto Warburg

Living an acidic lifestyle is one of the most harmful things you could possibly do to yourself. It results in long-term fatigue, chronic stress and fatal illnesses. Instead we must switch our pH levels from one that is more acidic to one that is more alkaline. Even if we eat acidic foods, and live stressful acidic lifestyles (stress increases acidity within the body), then we must ensure that the alkaline levels within our body are higher than the acidity levels in our system. As long as your alkaline intake is stronger than your acidity intake on a daily basis, then you should be healthier and more energetic.

How can we be more alkaline? Firstly, we should eat more greens, salads and vegetables. A great strategy is to eat your greens first whenever you have a meal otherwise we will fill up on other foods, and if we leave something, then it will likely be some vegetables or salad. We must mentally condition ourselves to always start by filling up on salads and vegetables. If the idea of eating salads every day does not really excite you, then you can make it taste richer by adding some feta cheese or halloumi or some pieces of fruit. Just be careful if you want to start adding things like sauces and croutons! Adding some lemon juice and apple cider vinegar not only makes your salad taste even better, but they will serve to supercharge your alkaline salad.

Secondly, in order to alkalise we must limit our intake of refined sugars (different variants of manufactured sugar) and most foods that are high in carbohydrates (as carbohydrates break down into simple sugars when being assimilated in the body). Reading the ingredient section for most of the foods that we eat can be alarming and demoralising as many of these acidic foods take on different, confusing names: high-fructose corn syrup (or any name with syrup in it for that mater!) as well as different names for sugar such as sucrose or saccharose. Additionally, be mindful of dairy, white flour and meat. Alcohol, and sugary fizzy drinks, contains extraordinary amounts of sugar, which is awful if we want to keep our body in an alkaline state. If regularly consumed, think about the low energy, negative thinking and potential illnesses that will arise if these are frequently consumed.

Thirdly, aim to exercise moderately every single day. Even if you have a gym workout already scheduled for that same day, embed a moderate and brief morning workout that takes just ten minutes! Mine includes bodyweight squats, push ups and crunches over and over. Sweating is a great way of detoxing the body and eliminating toxins from within. Keep the body moving and sweating as a way to keep the body pure and more alkaline. Be cautious with training intensely too often as overtraining creates acid in the body. As with everything, balance is necessary. Constantly evaluate how you feel, and let that dictate your physical exertion for the next day. Enjoying the sauna and steam rooms is another great way to reduce acid and the accumulation of toxins within the body. Cleanse. Cleanse. Cleanse.

Fourthly, drink lemon water, and water in general, copiously. Lemon juice is one of the easiest ways of alkalising the body. Ironically, most liquids with vinegar tend to increase acidity in the body except apple cider vinegar, which is a great way of alkalising the body as well as adding antioxidants and some amino acids. Lemon and apple cider vinegar water can be the best way to start your day, and to keep your pH level at the optimum level.

Fifthly, this one might seem surprising, but if stress induces acid, then we can partake in yoga and pilates, as a way of reducing stress and thus acidity within the body. Deep breathing in general is fantastic for cleansing the body and energising. These meditative exercises coincide to increase alkaline levels. Furthermore, even alternating hot and cold showers, or just cold showers alone for that matter, can be effective in increasing blood circulation, changing our breathing patterns and eliminating toxins in the body. Cold is the new hot!

A Captivating Lifestyle

"And yet, the only exciting life is the imaginary one." – Virginia Woolf

The key to true happiness in life is to surround ourselves with the people we love most, and to enjoy the process of achieving our deep desires and goals. We should frequently find time to do the things we most enjoy. We can only make others happy when we are happy with ourselves. Therefore, getting into great shape should not be seen as a negative in any way because we give more in many ways when we are happy and congruent with ourselves. The most selfish people in the world view themselves as victims. Those who are depressed are often very selfish indeed. Why? They only perceive things from their perspectives. They are only viewing things from their own point of view. Depression is therefore a result of having an overactive ego. One-way out of depression is to help and support others, and we can do that by being a role model: by becoming the people we really want to be. We must add value to the world by developing our skills, talents, knowledge, wealth and so on, so that people benefit from us mentally, emotionally and thus physically. Sometimes people view getting into shape as something that is purely about that person, but really the only real way to influence others in life is to set an example of what is possible and why.

An exciting life is all about constantly having something that we are immersed in because that is when we experience flow: a state of absolute focus and bliss. We can benefit from working on more than one goal at a time because momentum takes over, and we will begin to improve in all of these facets. We must ensure that we are preparing for the next step even before we have accomplished our current goal. People fall into depression when they have experienced a massive high, and then they decide to step back. Think about the stereotypical athlete who has an exciting, rich yet short career, and then he or she ends up depressed and squandering his or her finances. The same applies to astronauts: they achieve something that not many people will ever experience, and so when they return, they have nothing that even comes close to making them feel stimulated and significant. They then fall into depression. Even people who become rich after setting up and selling their business soon become depressed by just sitting around wasting their time. Boredom is a choice. Why do we experience boredom? We are bored because we either do not have enough energy to do things (poor lifestyle, eating habits, sleeping habits etc.), or we have not planned our lives well (we do not have meaningful goals or things that motivate us). Inertia and boredom are catalysts of depression. It is all about challenging ourselves, taking up new interests and expanding our current interests. This will indirectly affect our mental and emotional states, and thus the actions we do that support or hinder our physical goals.

"Extraordinary change can happen in your life, but it will take extraordinary people, extraordinary courage and extraordinary faith to believe that this won't be a repeat of your past." - Shannon L. Alder

Know your purpose; have a massive why, and make time to do the things that you love. This creates the kind of joy and pleasure needed to keep you positive, energetic and thus less prone to eating unhealthily. Happiness and health are intrinsically tied together. The more energy we have, the less we need external stimuli to change our state: unhealthy foods and drinks, addictions to drugs, alcohol and smoking that ruin us from the inside out. Energy enables us to think and move at our best consistently. It leads to greater efficiency, pleasure and ensures that we set high standards for ourselves in many avenues. Generally, the more we partake in fun and passionately driven activities, the more energy we have within. We must choose a job, career or business where, at the very least, there is more joy than displeasure. Doing things that we do not want to do, and doing these often every day, ruins our spirit. We have low energy, and therefore, people think things such as, "I don't know why I am always tired," or "How come I am even struggling to get basic tasks done?" Doing activities that, in our perception, do not add great value, coupled with an acidic eating regime, is a recipe for low energy and pain. Consistent low energy results in frequent sadness (as we do not understand why we feel so tired and incapable), which negatively affects our self-esteem, consequently resulting in depression. Acid leads to depression. Low energy and an acidic lifestyle will result in poor quality, low vibrational thoughts, emotions and incompetent actions. If we want to change our bodies, we must change our minds; if we want to change our minds, we must follow our passions, and partake in activities that we are passionate about.

Consider your current job, career or business. Take a moment to write down the type of activities you do on your average week. Decide whether each activity is more pleasurable or painful. Give each activity a percentage out of 100%: 0% meaning no pleasure and 100% meaning the highest level of joy. Create a table: on the left-hand side include all of the activities that bring you 50% or more joy and label that column, alkaline. Then on the right-hand side, write down everything that you scored under 50%, and label that column, acid. This may not be the case for everyone, but there is usually a link between the types of activities we do (how much pleasure or pain that derive from them), and what type of foods and drinks we consume. The more acidic our activities, the more acidic we are in our food and drink consumption. See how many activities you can minimise, eliminate or transfer from the acidic column. Moreover, contemplate how you can make the current alkaline-inducing activities even more alkaline!

Whilst sleep conspicuously helps us in terms of recovery and brain function, we want to live a life where we *want* to sleep less and be awake longer because our lives are so rich with meaning and quality states. This does not mean we should be sleeping less than five hours a day, but we should *want* to sleep as little as that because there is so much that we want to experience and do in order to attain our goals. We want to wake up feeling that we have a purpose, and we want to wake up feeling like this new day will take us closer to achieving our biggest goals. If you know today will be mediocre, then this will negatively affect your energy levels. Even if we work an average job, we can still wake up earlier and/or go to sleep later, so that we can do more flow-inducing activities or more important activities. We should be able to do something every single day that will improve our health, our relationships and our wealth. This ensures balance, high self-esteem and high energy.

The quality of our lives, and how much energy we have, is also down to whom we spend our time with. Sometimes we must spend time with people whom we do not necessarily like. However, in most instances, how much time we spend with people is really down to us. Distance yourself from negativity and fat-supporting people who directly or indirectly affect your body shape. If we do not like people at work, then we should get a new job. If we do not like how our friends treat us, then we should make new, positive friends. If we do not like our partner's energy, then we should consider our arrangements. These decisions are ultimately our choice. We want to spend time with people who have great energy because energy is infectious. We also want to avoid or limit our exposure to negative or low-energy people because we naturally lower our own energy and emotions in order to make others feel better. Again, it would be helpful to write a list of people in your life who have a more acidic or alkaline effect on us. Arguments, hostility, tension and all forms of abuse lead to negativity, and negativity results in bad momentum, which pervasively affects our eating and drinking habits. Keep your interactions with 'acidic people' brief and simple. Positive energy increases our energy levels whereas drama, arguments and conflict increase blood pressure, stress (acidity) and only bad decisions derive from negative energy.

"Energy is contagious, positive and negative alike. I will forever be mindful of what and who I am allowing into my space." - Alex Elle

Sleep

"Sleep is that golden chain that ties health and our bodies together."
– Thomas Dekker

We all need quality sleep. Quality sleep is actually more important than the quantity of sleep we have. Quality sleep means uninterrupted sleep. Sleeping more is not the answer, and it can actually make us less energetic. Regular sleeping patterns can help to lower stress levels, which will affect how much we eat and what we eat. Inconsistent levels of sleep can result in low energy, poor focus and greater agitation. These lead to increased hunger and a desperate need for energy. Anything done out of desperation will only enhance the acidity within us. Think about the things you do when desperate for energy. I am confident that they enhance acidity. Few hours of sleep every day is deleterious, but so is low quality sleep. Quality sleep can help us to maintain our existing weight. Quality sleep regulates the hormones that directly affect our appetite. Quality sleep will not only make us eat healthy amounts, but it will also prevent sugar cravings.

However, low quality sleep coupled with alcohol-fuelled nights can massively ruin hormone levels, energy, serotonin and relationships. All of the aforementioned consequences will lead to fat gain and reduced muscle mass. Good sleeping patterns has been shown to improve our moods. It keeps us consistent and congruent with who we really are whereas frequent low levels of quality sleep can make us short tempered and more prone to negative thinking and interactions. Moreover, quality sleep can help in terms of memory, mental sharpness and focus, which obviously results in higher self-confidence: we feel more capable, competent and communicative. Consider your recent sleeping patterns. What do you do before sleep, and what do you do upon waking? How do they support or ruin your alkaline levels and quality of sleep?

Supplements

We must provide the body with what it needs in order to think and move as best as we can. I am not advocating what supplements you should take. I will simply outline what I personally use, and I will explain the benefits of these supplements. Firstly, I consume fish oils daily. Fish oils can contribute to weight loss. It can also reduce inflammation. Moreover, it can potentially improve bone health and support joints. Secondly, I benefit tremendously from supplementing with vitamin D (especially necessary if you live in the UK!), as it can protect our bones whilst helping to prevent many bone diseases. It makes sense, but vitamin D can help to improve potential seasonal sadness, as it may affect the activity of serotonin. Additionally, it can help to prevent cognitive decline, and serious illnesses. Thirdly, I like to take ZMA (zinc, magnesium and vitamin B6), but you can consume them individually if you prefer. The essential mineral, zinc, helps with muscle growth and recovery. Magnesium, another essential mineral, supports the function of our cardiovascular system and our bone health. Moreover, it can support heart health, support calcium absorption and prevent diabetes. Combined, these essential minerals can build muscle size whilst also supporting fat loss. Vitamin B complex supplementation can reduce stress whilst boosting our moods. It may also reduce anxiety and depression. Additionally, it functions to boost energy levels, and we know how high levels of energy affect our eating and drinking habits. These are the essentials that I use in order to increase my energy and wellbeing.

Circumventing Inertia

"The real key is to live in an environment where the mind feels free to choose the right thing instead of being compelled by habit and inertia to choose the wrong thing." – Deepak Chopra

No one is powerful when tired. People simply cannot perform well, or even think positively, if they are tired. The more energy we have, the more positive and vibrant we feel. This is why it is so important to sleep, eat and exercise well. Here is a strategy to use when we feel exhausted. Firstly, we need to dramatically change our physiology, so we must literally do the opposite to what we do when we are exhausted: how do you prepare yourself mentally and physically before taking part in a competition? How do you stretch? Do you beat your chest or make a fist with your hand? We associate these gestures with alertness and readiness. They instinctively have the same effect even if we are about to go into a meeting or start reading extensively. Secondly, we must focus on our breathing. What is its speed? How long and deep do we inhale and exhale? Again do the exact opposite. Take several vigorous breaths. Breathe inwards with velocity, and blow out every bit of breath with fervour and determination. Make your exhale last longer than the inhale. If we have an anchor set (a movement we have conditioned by associating feelings of power and confidence with that gesture), now would be a good time to use it. We should now feel more vigilant and active.

Reward Yourself

Last but not least, we can increase our energy levels in the long term by celebrating and rewarding ourselves every time we achieve something. This can be on a small scale like celebrating eating healthily for a week or longer by enjoying an unrestricted meal with family and friends. We can also benefit from celebrating larger successes in our personal and professional lives by going on holidays, purchasing material goods or looking after our bodies in the form of treatments and so on. We want to create the feeling that we are always succeeding, and moving closer to the attainment of our major goals in life. It helps to keep us motivated to achieve more whilst also providing us with some variety which is often needed due to the regimented and disciplined lives we need to support our health and physical shapes. Without these rewards, we can become fatigued and we may feel like we are never getting anywhere (when really we are) because we question why we sacrifice things more and more. This is why we all need breaks every now and then whether it is a break for two hours or a weekend. However, aim to keep yourself busy, motivated and excited as often as possible because that is how we build momentum and avoid boredom (negativity and poor eating).

"Everything around is made up of energy. To attract positive things in your life, start by giving off positive energy." - Anonymous

Chapter 8 - The Shift

"The only person you are destined to become is the person you decide to be." - Ralph Waldo Emerson

The shift is all about creating an incredible life, which will massively affect our bodies. The happier and more successful we feel, the more we love and care about ourselves. We become even more focused on looking after our health and bodies because we want to live as long as possible, and we want to feel as though we can accomplish anything we want, which includes physical goals. This section is really about maximizing your potential mentally, so that you can create the kind of quality life that you want. Your mentality and emotions will determine your overall physical shape; it is a long-term strategy that will keep you in great physical shape rather than just wanting to look great now because you are single or because it is your 'ego' phase and so on. We want to rewire our lives, so that we feel happy and healthy for the rest of our lives regardless of what happens to our metabolism as we age.

Everything happens for a reason. There is a reason why you have come across this book now. What happens to us is a culmination of the type of energy we bring forward, and the energy of other people's thoughts and feelings about us. This is why we must seek to find only good things coming into our lives. There is no right or wrong path. We certainly control our own overall destiny. We just need to steady the ship if things are not going well for many people around us. If we listen and feel enough positivity, then we can act in positive ways to get us out of pernicious predicaments. Of course we can affect the direction and experiences in our lives. However, we must view the wider picture, and not become disheartened if we are not where we currently wish to be. Energies have not been brought together yet. We attract what happens in our lives. Planning and attracting nice things to happen to us are important, but there is more to it than that. We must also undertake the necessary action to accomplish our goals. We must be willing to meet the universe half way.

We all have our own individual energy force. The area we inhabit has some sort of metaphorical circle around us that exudes our energy. When we encounter someone, we are interacting with his or her energy. Have you ever met someone, and for some weird reason you had a sense of exactly how they are for better or worse? Have you ever looked somewhere and caught someone staring at you? What was that? Your antenna was instinctively aware that someone else's gaze and focus was on you. Does it stop here? Are there other energetic fields available to access, which we simply cannot detect? There is a sort of invisible detection that we all have. It is worth considering what kind of energy we have, what it attracts, and what types of people (energies) we interact with daily. Low vibrations will reduce the quality of our vibrations; high, powerful, loving vibrations can uplift and inspire our energy and vice versa. Maybe there is something to the saying, fake it until we make it. If we act as though we have everything that we desire, including an amazing body, which we all should feel anyway, then we will be in a place to attract like-minded people who have the skills, resources and experience we can learn from.

Positive thoughts occur more often when we have great mental and physical energy; negative thoughts creep up on us when we are most tired. These moments can be greatly reduced, but, to a degree, they are also inevitable: what comes up must come down. Fortunately, we can live our lives generally with great energy, depending upon how we live and what habits we employ daily. Boredom and tiredness are intertwined, which reveals the power of being in flow as much as possible. Do you sometimes have strong energy, but when it dawns on you that you have to complete a laborious task, suddenly you lack that physical and mental capacity? Fortunately, we know some techniques to apply now to change our state. We also understand how our minds work better now, and so we can preempt that we will suddenly get tired when we get to our desk etc. We know how our own minds try to trick us.

Instead, we can use our disappointments to make ourselves even better. They can ignite our desire to get better, stronger, smarter, sexier and thus, ironically, more self-assured. Life comes down to how much fight we have in us. This is why we all love the story of the underdog who ends up winning: we know that it can be done if we just apply ourselves and believe in ourselves. If we are to fight in life, we must have enough energy to drive us through challenging moments. We die and pass on when we eventually lose the fight in this dimension. The happiest and most successful people in life are those who see abundance and opportunity everywhere. It is mightily significant to have high self-esteem. Self-esteem and confidence are different: confidence refers to knowing our ability and strengths within a given activity whereas self-esteem refers to how much love and appreciation we have for ourselves generally (whether we are doing well or 'badly' at something). How can we build self-esteem? Love how we are now. Yes, we can always get better at things, but know that we are enough just the way we are right now. Everyone is imperfect, and the more we seek perfection (unless we are humble in our pursuit), then the more imbalanced and thus disturbed we will become.

There are three priorities we should all seek to constantly improve if we are to live balanced and incredible lives. Firstly, we must prioritise our health. We must continuously look to improve our health in a multitude of ways: ensure that we sleep well; reduce stress by partaking in our favourite activities often; eat quality, nutrient-dense foods 90% of the time; drink plenty of water; consume fundamental supplements (fish oils, vitamin D, zinc and magnesium); have sex often; be active (don't always look to park closest to your destination for instance; train at least three times per week); drink and eat greens! These health rules will make us feel lighter, more energetic, and we will not incur as much mental and physical pain as we grow older. The way we eat and drink now will be felt ten years from now. Secondly, our relationships should always take precedence. It is wise to only have a small circle of people with whom we trust with anything and everything. Make time for them! Share, communicate, laugh and give as much as we can with these wonderful people whether they are family or friends. Our relationships are often like muscles: if we do not put effort in, then our relationships will 'atrophy.' Thirdly, our wealth is key. Regardless of our beliefs, and how we perceive money, let us be honest. Money is very important to us all. We will incur problems whether we are rich or poor; it is easier to face our problems if we are a strong financial position. It is just the world we live in, and so it is a game we must learn to play well. Consistently reflect on your business, career and assets. Go on courses, research profusely, and take action! The animal kingdom is naturally determined by survival of the fittest; they rise to the top based on strength and size. Humans, however, are different. Our version of survival of the fittest is down to how much wealth we accrue. It is the nature of the beast (no pun intended)!

Consistently reflect upon these three priorities. Monthly, give yourself a score out of ten for how well you are doing in each department (ten being incredible and zero being atrocious), and take certain actions depending on which one has been lacking recently. This ensures balance, and a clear mind, which will always benefit our bodies. If we are doing well in these three areas, then we tend to exude robust energy. We will attract more. Things are never as easy as they seem, and things are never as hard as they seem. Bare this in mind, and we will not incur as many disappointments or surprises in our lives.

The Present Moment

"Do not dwell in the past, do not dream of the future, concentrate the mind on the present moment." - Buddha

Why spend time dwelling on the past when it is over? Why worry about the distant future when it is unknown? Instead primarily focus on the present moment, as this is the moment we can enjoy and make the most occur. Problems are continuous and never lacking. We will always have problems; even the most spiritual, peaceful and happy of us have problems. The key is how we deal with these problems, and what we associate with them. Some problems are necessary, healthy and good: how can we increase profits so that they are higher than last year's? This is a great problem! However, other problems are intoxicating, and they could poison us within if we allow its pervasive and insidious nature to pulse through our veins and literally destroy our cells through stress over time. Really, all we ever really have is the present moment. Perceive every day as though it is a mini life: be productive; see or talk to the ones you love; make some time for your favourite hobby and interest; give to others (working on your business or career). Make every single day the most productive, giving and loving day of your life.

"If you abandon the present moment you cannot live the moments of your daily life deeply." – Thich Nhat Hanh

Many unhappy people are too busy focusing on their past especially things that went wrong or pondering how good things were lost. Conversely, there are those who focus purely on the future. The only problem with this is that whilst our future will inevitably improve as a result, we are never actually satisfied because we are never actually fully living in the present moment. The best approach is to alternate between, frequently but briefly, thinking about the future (in the form of planning and setting goals, and thinking long-term about things) whilst also living in the present, so we can enjoy where we are now and really experience life in its most natural form: being present in the moment.

We must believe that we are only as good as we are meant to be right now. It does not matter if we were once rich or famous or happy or driven or once had a great body. What are we like right now? This belief will ensure that we challenge ourselves, and live in the present moment as opposed to nostalgically dwelling on what once was. This is how people become depressed: they actually oscillate mentally between the past and their present helplessness rather than focusing on the present and planning their future optimistically. Consider how often you live in the present moment. Why might we be so attached to events in the past? How can we move forward? Why must we move forward?

Our minds are often work on autopilot. This is when the subconscious takes over. This is where learned routines, in terms of thought and feelings, circulate and continue our underlying belief systems: "How do I look?" "What do others think of me?" "Why do I make these mistakes?"

"Why can't I meet someone amazing?" "I don't have enough money." "I need more friends and attention." The mind is left to wander, and it reverts to what it knows. It can be influenced by our deep desires and fears. These can definitely be changed if we are self-reflective, persistent and catch ourselves when we are about to fall into the same trap. If we keep replaying things over and over again in our mind, then we will manifest the same result in a slightly different context. We will remain fixed with the same personality we have right now, and that cannot happen if we need to massively change out lives: we have to change who we are (our thoughts, emotions and actions must change). There must be a shift.

Our Reactions

"A positive attitude causes a chain reaction of positive thoughts, events and outcomes. It is a catalyst and it sparks extraordinary results."
– Wade Boggs

If we are washing the dishes, and we smash a glass, then what are our reactions? While this seems trivial and fruitless, it actually demonstrates our natural emotions when things do not go our way, and when we have made a mistake. How do we respond? "Why am I so clumsy?" "Why am I so stupid?" "See, this is what happens when my wife stresses me out!" Hopefully you have a more appeasing response: "It happens sometimes." "We aren't perfect." "Well if that's the worst thing that happens to me this month, then I am fortunate." One person begins to shout and blame others or themselves while another remains serene and loving. One says, "This happened because no one helps me" while the other says, "What a shame, I guess I better slow down" or "That was my mistake; I better take it easy for now." This all comes down to how we treat ourselves. It reflects our self-esteem. It reveals whether we are a 'victim,' or if we take responsibility. These reactions are closely connected to how we appease ourselves or stress ourselves, which definitely affects our physical aspirations.

Do we take responsibility for our actions, or do we use an external force as an excuse? A controversial moment such as this may appear innocuous, but this reaction enhances an emotion, and it can have a domino effect on how many other events unfold during the day. A simple thought ("I am stupid," or "It is all right; I forgive myself"), influences our emotions (feeling angry or loving), which then results in a behavioural change (not taking part in such useful activities for fear of failure, or an appreciation that sometimes things do not go our way, but we must keep doing our best). This seemingly insignificant pattern, over time, leads to a greater scenario with larger ramifications: making an error at work; having an argument with a loved one; even how we react when approaching someone of the opposite sex for the first time. Even if the context is different, the pattern is the same! These reactions and patterns not only determine our destiny, they also deeply affect how we interact and share emotions with others. We not only set up positive or negative structures within ourselves, but we also embed these in others (that is if they choose to agree with us or disassociate themselves). We all now know that positivity, optimism and high energy are essential for the development of an incredible body.

Our reactions to externals are indicative of our internal representations: whether we have healthy and positive reactions or defensive and negative ones. The external influences the internal, and the internal influences the external. This back and forth cycle ascertains how we perceive and interpret things. Listen to the following words. What thoughts or emotions come to mind when you hear them? Depression... Rich... Pain... Interest... Love... The first image, thought or emotion that comes to mind must be analysed and evaluated. This is the connection that we make to the word at this present moment. If we are unhappy with the result, and can see the negative connotations that we make, then do not be disheartened as this can be changed. We simply have to practice reconditioning the image and word interconnections. Here is another example: is there a particular song that reminds you of a past or present lover? This association can be changed if we wish. It is all about running the song over and over again, but thinking of something completely different with great emotional intensity. This is one way of mitigating our current associations to things. We must understand ourselves well enough, and in a way, plan our reactions to things just in case we have to go through that experience. The more prepared we are, the more options we have. We not only need to stay one step ahead of our competition; we also need to stay one step ahead of ourselves.

Our Patterns

"Patterns of repetition govern each day, week, year, and lifetime... But I say these habits are sacred because they give deliberate structure to our lives. Structure gives us a sense of security."
– Robert Fulghum

What things do we do repetitiously every day? What do we think about when we physically do them? The more we think about something when in mild trance-like states (exercising, washing dishes, cleaning the house, reading, playing computer games etc.), the stronger the associations become. If we brush our teeth, and think about how difficult our day will be, then do not be surprised why we do not enjoy brushing our teeth! If we experience mental entropy and negative thoughts whilst driving, then we will not enjoy the process of driving in the future. If we talk about negative and depressing issues, then we give power and energy to them. Become conscious of your thoughts, and how topics move from one to the next in your mind and why. See if you can understand the psychological connections you make. For example, we may go from thinking about our ex partner to thinking about a boss we hated to then thinking about the business we are thinking of launching. Firstly, what connection is there? We have linked them all to failure or pain. Secondly, we have presupposed that the possible business would be damaging to us, and a complete failure. It can be very revealing. We must be mindful of what we think about when we are physically doing things. With repetition this becomes powerful and strengthened.

Firstly, we can change negative trances by installing a more positive method of mental relaxation: exercise, yoga, sport, reading, writing, playing music and so on. Secondly, we can also consciously work on rewiring our associations by using enough intense positive and powerful statements and questions to uplift, motivate and overwhelm the negative, biological voice that operates within all of us. Our habits condition our daily lives, which reinforces our identity. Sometimes we need a different experience to trigger new patterns: the link between our thoughts, emotions and actions (our character).

Our Reality

"You know you're in love when you can't fall asleep because reality is finally better than your dreams." – Dr. Seuss

What we believe will become our reality. If we believe in Islamic practices, then we are right. If we believe in Christianity, then we are right. If we believe in trust, then we are right. Whatever we believe to be the truth, the core of our existence, then we are right. Our internalisation is our truth. We create our energy, our divinity, and our effects on others. Our energy infects others, and meshes with the universe's energy to affect others one way or another. If we believe it, so it shall be. Unfortunately, or fortunately, people become rigid and stubborn in their thoughts and beliefs, which is perilous to the self: we limit what we can think, experience and share. We can only see from our eyes this way, and even if we believe in a wider cause, it is the ego that rears its ugly face whenever we undermine or belittle another's beliefs. The paradox is that we are always complete, yet whenever we stop learning and challenging ourselves, we metaphorically and spiritually die. We must be flexible in our beliefs, not necessarily docile and malleable, but capable of change. Anyone who remains the same no longer fits in today's ever-changing world. If we are inflexible, we will not progress. We must be like water. Do not work against what is natural. We all have a purpose, and an ability to profoundly affect others. We must decide what our ideal selves are, and make decisions based on these promising self-prototypes.

Physical muscles grow when they are pushed beyond its 'boundaries.' The same exact principle applies to the mind and our willpower. To break through we must become uncomfortable. Unfortunately, this is often when people stop, and they feel helpless. This is often when procrastination and excuse making comes into play. No character is being built when people do not break through. A weak character is a consequence of weak thoughts and weak standards. How do we know when we have broken through a metaphorical barrier? What is it that we always, or frequently, say to ourselves when we reach the peak of something difficult? "I can't swim another lap." "If I fail, I'll look stupid." "I've never been able to do it before." "I'm just not good at it." "This is enough for me." In these instances, the key words are obvious: "Can't," "stupid," "never," "not good," and so on. We must condition ourselves, so that when we reach these points, we say something more inspiring and uplifting. The powerful words, "I am" must be followed with whatever positive phrases we want. Now that we are conscious of what we say when in these situations, we must apply a vibrant image or clip of success in our minds, and affirm using this chosen positive phrase over and over: "I am successful" "I am going to accomplish this" or even better, "I have already accomplished this," or "I deserve this." All we need to focus on is taking just one step at a time.

If we are struggling to tackle something challenging, then we should begin something even harder than what we already have as a barrier to our progression. Doing something even more dangerous or challenging brilliantly utilises the power of contrast. The initial task does not seem as daunting now. For example, if you are anxious about attending a new gym class for whatever reason, then sign up for a hardcore and intense training program. Even so, things always have a way of working out, if we can learn to have faith and work on what we value. Yes, we can dictate our journeys, but to achieve this poetically, we must accept all that happens in our lives. Things can always have a beautiful spin to them (context reframing) if we so choose to give it one.

We all have thresholds for different things. Some thresholds are higher than others, and this is usually influenced by our priorities. The way to grow is to always place demands on these thresholds, always pushing slightly more each time until our previous threshold is no longer a barrier, and we can push further, experience newer, and, thus, be happier. Mental and physical health is achieved by continuous growth in areas that we value. Health, and a six-pack, is not something we will just attain one day, like a possession. Even if we think we will be permanently happy if we just had a great body, and never had to train or eat well again, we would be wrong. Boredom, complacency and the subsequent negative thoughts will soon seep into our extra freedom unless we find new inspiring activities. We must constantly challenge and break barriers to sustain true contentment and inner peace.

Think about the physical journey we most often make: usually to a workplace, relative's house or friend's place. What we will notice is that our minds go on autopilot due to the familiarity of the scenery and routine. This creates comfort and relaxation, but will rarely ever fill us with new thoughts. However, when we explore an 'unfamiliar journey,' our minds operate differently, often with chaos and randomness, and a whole range of extreme thoughts and emotions may pervade our fluency. Where there is chaos, there is a chance to create something new: a new belief. A challenge to customary thinking begins. This analogy is just how we live our own lives. We become complacent and unnecessarily comfortable. It is impossible to grow, progress and experience anew unless we travel down a different path (both physically and mentally).

Breakthrough

"He who desires but acts not breeds pestilence." - William Blake

We will never change and take control of our lives unless we have built enough emotional strength to be resilient. Change can happen in an instant. It only takes one moment or event to push us pass our threshold: when we have had enough of something, and we know we must make a change. The intensity of this emotion has broken our patterns, and we are ready to perceive anew. Something switches inside. Our internal language patterns change, our feelings change and a new belief (new found certainty) is set in motion. These changes not only affect how we are in relation to that specific activity, but it also pervades into other elements. Everything is connected in one way or another. Consider how improving your career might affect your physical body. Consider how making your major relationships stronger and more positive might affect your physical body.

Unfortunately, many people have different thresholds, which are linked to their blueprints. For example, one person may only need to gain four pounds of fat in order to think that enough is enough, and they must regain their focus and lose weight whereas another person will need to gain say twenty pounds of fat in order to reach their threshold. We have thresholds for everything in life, and the quality of our lives in based on the standards we set: the quality of our blueprints. The higher our blueprints are, the shorter our thresholds become. We can flip the switch (reaching our threshold) more quickly, and change when problems start early rather than waiting, coming up with excuses and then struggling even more because we are so far behind. Consider the blueprints you have as it relates to your relationships, your health and your wealth. Could these be set higher? What is your threshold until you look to improve a relationship or your health or your wealth? What has to happen? Now is the time to recondition yourself, and breakthrough to the next level.

Resilience

"The more you sweat in practice, the less you bleed in battle." – Unknown Author

If we are to improve the quality of our health and bodies, then we will need to overcome internal and external challenges. Every single time we have to do something new or unfamiliar, we will meet resistance in the form of unhelpful negative thoughts. The key to circumventing this is proactivity and anticipation. We must be able to predict some of the thoughts and feelings we will evoke when encountering the unknown. If we are going to a job interview, we must anticipate that we will feel incapable or stressed at some point during the process, which is oftentimes in the lead up to the actual event: "I just don't think I have all the skills needed yet, so I should really just cancel the interview and attempt this when I am definitely ready." The problem is we will never be completely ready! If we are about to go on a first date, anticipate that we will feel like the date is not worth going to: "What is the point of going on that date today? I mean we might not even connect that well. Plus, there are things I need to do. We can go out another time." The problem is if we do not have the urgency to meet now, when feelings and information are new and interesting, then when will you actually meet? The same applies to our health: we will often question why we are eating so healthily or why we must gym again this week, and so we must have mechanisms in place to always push us forward in moments of uncertainty. Be ready for your negative talk, and have positive affirmations ready to keep you on track.

Do not make promises to yourself, or others, if you know you cannot keep them. Every time we do not follow through with something we really want to do, or something we know we should do, we trust ourselves less and less, and we begin to doubt ourselves more and more. Not being able to live up to our promises, such as not going to the gym class you intended on going to, will pervade into other promises that you have made: losing ten pounds of fat. It ruins the congruency within us. The next time we genuinely think to ourselves, "Right, I have to start this diet today. Enough is enough!" we will have a subsequent thought that will say, "Who are you kidding. You never follow through." We now begin to identify ourselves as someone who talks, but does not execute. What does this do to our self-belief? This negativity then manifests itself within other areas of our lives as we have now created a limiting belief. The label, "I am someone who does not follow through" then rears its ugly head whenever we want to travel the world or start up a business or create a work of art or attempt another healthy eating plan in the future and so on.

"Everything you attract into your life is a reflection of the story you believe and keep telling yourself." – Farshad Asl

What we think about proliferates. What we say, and the kind of words we use internally, will dictate our experience. We must focus on how emotive, extreme and hyperbolic our vocabulary actually is at times. For example, was that workout fun or onerous? Was your performance all right or spectacular? Was the event fantastic or decent? Are you feeling fine or incredible? This is even more important when we face adversity. When in a pressurised, precarious or tense position, the language we use is vital. Was the environment hostile or uncomfortable? Was the argument vicious or insensitive? Was your partner unkind or brutal? The vocabulary we use cuts off our possibilities and limits our options. For instance, if we are losing in a competition, we could communicate with ourselves in many ways. Limiting and negative questions would be: "This is usually when we fall apart. Why does it always happen?" whereas promising and optimistic language sounds like, "We will keep moving forward because we are more talented than them. They will break." We can condition how we respond in moments of uncertainty because of the beliefs that we have built about ourselves: "I never stop until I get the job done," or "I always find a way." The more we repeat these with intense emotions, the more they become automatic whenever we are in difficult situations. We need a wealth of positivity and fortitude because it is human nature to consider things when we are uncomfortable, and when we can choose immediate gratification (not going gym or eating poorly) above our long-term goals.

Abundance

"Abundance is not something we acquire. It is something we tune into."
- Wayne Dyer

People often eat unhealthily when they think a certain type of food will not be there for long. Scarcity is a very powerful tool that businesses use on us, and that we often use on ourselves. This sense of scarcity is linked to deeper limiting thinking across all levels. This is why many people always finish the food on their plate. They were taught to eat like this out of fear usually from their parents: there is not enough in the world or even for us. Make it a rule to never finish eating every last bit on your plate; you are not allowed to leave salad and vegetables though! Some believe in scarcity: they think that there is not enough money in the world; they think that there are not enough interesting people who will want them; they believe that there are not enough people out there who will like them for who they are etc. We attract what we think about most frequently, and we attract what we feel most frequently. All we need to do is remain focused on our goals, plan well and keep mentally and physically healthy.

In stark contrast, there are those who believe in abundance: they believe that they can attract as much money, potential partners and friends as they wish.

Whatever you truly believe to be the truth, will become your reality, so why not just choose to believe in the best possible things? This mentality must be cultivated. If we want to attract anything we want, then the shift must take place across all areas. There is enough of everything that we want in the world, and if we believe otherwise, then we have been falsely conditioned. We must be congruent with our beliefs. Begin to cultivate the belief that you can have whatever you desire. You can have a great body, yet do excellently at work, and yet raise a strong, happy family. It is possible when we believe, and thus attract, abundance. Contemplate your perceptions about what you genuinely think you can become in all key areas of your life: this is what you think your potential is, which should be limitless. Also, contemplate what you think cannot be done. Write these down and write down why you think they cannot be achieved. Cross these excuses out one at a time by replacing them with things that you can, and will, do from now on.

Momentum

"A positive attitude causes a chain reaction of positive thoughts, events and outcomes. It is a catalyst and it sparks extraordinary results."
– Wade Boggs

When we want to be successful at something, we must also continue to improve upon our current strengths, as our successes in these existing avenues can positively affect our current weaknesses also. Things may seem unrelated, but as with much in life, they are oftentimes interconnected. If we want to increase our success at work, then we can take the pressure off by performing well in the gym; if we want to improve the quality of our relationships, then we can improve upon our interests (whether it is art, writing, sports and so on). Build success upon success. Develop that winning mentality. I have personally noticed a link within my own life: the more I give to my family, and those who are more vulnerable in the world, the more money I attract and move toward; the more money I accumulate, the easier it is for me to eat healthily and train intelligently. These improvements work together to really improve my self-esteem. We must develop the belief that we will always find a way to succeed. This builds character. Do what you want to do because that is the only way you will truly accept and love yourself. This even works with hobbies: if we give great devotion to an interest, such as swimming, then we can diversify our exercise regime by incorporating martial arts or football or golf. The change in perception allows us to take a step back from our main goal, in this instance swimming, whilst allowing us to enjoy another similarly related interest. It can take the form of an enjoyable distraction, and take away any tension associated with what we initially want to take precedence.

There is no particular correct way of doing things in life. We all have different paths and admirable qualities whether discernible or latent. The key to success is momentum. Momentum is the ability to transfer the passion and enthusiasm generated from one success into another. One way of doing this is by identifying the strategy that worked well in one area and using it, in one way or another, in another area. For example, what makes you good at your job? One factor might be that you are always consistent. Consistency is also required to maintain a strong and healthy body. What makes your relationships so powerful and strong? It might be your honesty. Honesty is also needed with yourself if you are not to by into the excuses that we can sometimes make when we do not feel like going to the gym or eating healthily. How does a business become very lucrative? Great marketing and branding helps of course. Well we will also need to display our bodies often and develop a great reputation that we are dedicated to losing fat. This transparency, and the constant physical reminders, can keep us on track. We can use this positivity and success as leverage. Unfortunately, there are all types of obstacles waiting to destroy this momentum such as a jealous friend, a stressful spouse, noisy and needy children, the monotony of a suppressing job and so forth. We must be proactive enough to understand that obstacles will arise; we must anticipate them, and have a positive comeback ready when they eventually appear.

Stability

"So much of what is best in us is bound up in our love of family, that it remains the measure of our stability because it measures our sense of loyalty. All other pacts of love or fear derive from it and are modeled upon it." - Haniel Long

Stability is a fundamental feature that we all need in order to feel grounded. Stability fills us with total clarity and reassurance, so that we can really make the most of our potential. Strong ethics breed stability. Our rituals and belief systems drive stability. Stability is essential for us to have the foundations in place to thrive and be happy. We cannot really focus on losing fat and looking amazing if we have more fundamental concerns. These must be addressed first otherwise our physical improvements simply will not last very long. Hence why people often lose a few pounds on a diet, and then end up not only gaining it all back, but even a little more than before! Maslow's hierarchy of needs brilliantly exemplifies the stages we must surmount one step at a time. Firstly, according to Maslow, our physiological needs must be met (shelter, food, warmth, sleep etc.) if we are able to function properly at all. We cannot think straight if we need to go to the toilet. We cannot think straight if we are really hungry. We cannot think straight if we are massively sleep deprived. We must have these basic needs met, so that we have the energy and focus needed to excel.

Secondly, we must all feel safe. If we feel threatened emotionally or physically, whether in a specific moment or over a certain period of time, then we can never truly maximise our potential. If we are excessively concerned about our health and wellbeing, then we cannot press forward. Everything we do is defensive and constrained rather than confident and assertive. The same applies if we have an illness. Feeling unsafe breeds psychic entropy. We desperately need order and control in order to feel secure. Thirdly, we need to feel a sense of belonging. We must feel connected to people, or at least ourselves, if we are to feel loved, appreciated and accepted. We must feel that we are part of a troop. Our main troop should always be our family. If we are not close with family, then we must seek this troop in the form of our closest friends. If this is not possible, then maybe we can build a troop at our workplace. By troop, we are referring to having absolute trust and unconditional love for the members within this close community. If we feel loved and connected, then we begin to make better choices, but if we do not, then we tend to be more impulsive and erratic in our actions. This does not help our health and six-pack goals!

Fourthly, only once we have stability in our lives, in the form of the previous three phases, then we can really develop our self-esteem. We can begin to explore new avenues, challenge our abilities and feel a sense of significance and power. This is the stage where we wish to excel in terms of our careers. We feel successful at this stage. Fifthly, we can become self-actualised, which is all about giving and growing as a person. We are so full inside that we wish to teach, share and give what we have in terms of our knowledge, experiences, wealth and so on. Is it possible that we can skip steps? For example, if we act as though we are self-actualised (by giving in all of these various forms), then will that also develop our self-esteem, which can make us feel more loved and connected to others, which can make us feel safer, allowing us to cure our inner and physical ailments (to an extent), and thus feel physiologically safer because we have shifted our perspective? I think so. We should then look to add value, give and share as much as we can in all avenues if we are to truly feel powerful, happy and successful. The more valued we feel, the more we care about our health and reputation, which relates to our appearance of course.

Have you ever given up on a goal? We all had something we wanted to achieve, but somewhere along the way our beliefs could only take us so far. We became distracted, we procrastinated and we lowered our expectations. We gave in, and we gave up. This is a natural human experience, but it should be unacceptable as of now. We are not victims regardless of what challenging or traumatic experiences we have endured. The moment we claim to be a victim is the moment we relinquish any form of responsibility. Leaders are responsible. Winners are responsible. The weak come up with excuses. The weak point at everyone except themselves. Every struggle encountered has been part of our journey. We all have our own destinies and purposes on earth. The most disappointing thing in life is that many of us do not manage to remove the dirt that covers the gold within us. We all have a light within us, yet, for many, our light goes unnoticed. It remains suppressed and subjugated for one reason or another: our upbringing and embedded limiting beliefs; our desire to fit in with our peers, thereby forcing us to lower our standards; we have listened to negative stories from others about why and how we will never make it. However, it is us who chose to listen. We chose to restrict ourselves. Fortunately, this does not have to be the case any longer.

As we grow older, changing our habits become increasingly more challenging, as we physically and mentally become more rigid and inflexible. We become more hopeless due to our overriding fear; we succumb to our forthcoming departure from the physical world and many lose their sense of purpose. Simply accepting that we cannot change, however, illustrates that we have a fixed limiting belief. It is never too late to change. All we ever have is our present moments. Why choose to spend these present moments immersed in our worries and limited thoughts? Make a choice. I am reminded of a powerful ending of a renowned play: *The Death of Ivan Ilyich* by Tolstoy. The play is based on the protagonist's imminent death: he has lived a life of mediocrity; he has suffered from awful personal and financial matters as well as horrible relationships. In the final few moments of his life, he asks one spine-tingling question that provokes great thought. Ivan Ilyich says, "What *if my whole life* has been wrong?" We do not want to have any regrets when our time in this realm is over. This is why we must set high standards for our physical conditions, hold ourselves to account and live by our own beliefs and not the crippling beliefs others thrust upon us.

Our House

Our foundations must be strong otherwise our 'house' or 'tree' can neither be built, nor can it grow to its maximum potential. We can still accomplish some magnificent things, but more often than not, these will be lost as a result of not having the foundations in place to keep us strong. A building is not strong because it looks unique or powerful; it is only strong if it was built properly from the bottom. A house (our lives) is not just built on top of land: builders must dig deep into the ground to ensure that the foundations are strong before any bricks become visible on top of the surface. Unfortunately, many people neglect the foundations of their lives because it is not pretty, or because it is the hardest part to work on (the mind). They prefer to see results quickly due to sheer impatience. We look at an athlete's impeccable body, and we focus only on what we see. We look at the wealth of the businesswoman, and focus purely on what she has. We do not see the unattractive things that these successful people must do in order to become outstanding in their fields.

As the saying goes, Rome was not built in a day. The impatient house owners jump ahead, and focus on the elaborate, luxurious furniture inside, the magnificent windows, the gigantic television and so on. One day the house will collapse. Why? The foundations were not strong enough to begin with. The structure of the building was neglected. Our buildings (bodies) will not remain strong and lean if we think in the short term. Our buildings will not last if they are neglected. We must focus on what matters: our priorities. We may have beautiful and gorgeous things within the house, but these will be shattered if the entire building, our minds, collapses. Our belief systems are the roots of our 'garden's tree,' or the foundations of our 'house.' If we have any limiting beliefs, rigid fixations and traumatising memories from our childhoods that have not been dealt with, then there is no point concentrating purely on the future. We will all incur problems and obstacles in life, and we will not have the foundations in place to effectively deal with life's issues unless these underlying issues are addressed. We must make peace with our past. We must condition ourselves. Without a flexible mindset, integrated with strong, assertive belief systems, we will mentally break every time we face a real challenge; make no mistake about it, staying in great physical shape is a real challenge for all.

Patience

"Patience, persistence and perspiration make an unbeatable combination for success." – Napoleon Hill

The information age is truly overwhelming yet incredible. Never before have we had the ability to share ideas, communicate and eradicate many problems in the world. While many wondrous things have arisen, there are also several problems that stem from today's innovative and flexible nature where things are changing exponentially and uncontrollably. Depression experienced by youngsters and adolescents are at an all-time high. People are accustomed to getting what they want at the click of a button, but with this, patience greatly diminishes. People live busy, hectic lives where distractions are here, there and everywhere. People lose their concentration far too easily, and they give up on things more quickly simply because it takes too much time and energy. This could be one reason why we see such a high divorce rate: people lose their patience with their partners more readily, and it is incredibly easy to meet another partner these days. Amongst all of this chaos, it is down to us to remain in control. This can be achieved by greatly reducing our exposure to excessive news and drama both publicly and in our personal lives. Ensure that you have some time away from your phone and its distractions. It provides much needed time to reflect, relax and to let the mind calm down: all facets required for fat loss and muscle development.

Overcoming an obstacle, in any area, creates the clarity, optimism and resolve needed to also improve our physical shape. We are happy when we are progressing. Once we think that we have achieved it all, then boredom and complacency set in. We now know that depression is not far away either at this stage. We are never the finished article, and we should appreciate this. The more we reduce and control our fears, the more confident and impregnable we shall become. It is like searching for treasure. The more you *try* to achieve something, the harder it will be to attain. Everything must flow. Peace and harmony within will cultivate success. The earth orbits the sun and the moon orbits the earth. View your success as a natural transition based on the effort, knowledge and drive you are currently utilising and developing.

Embracing Silence

"All of humanity's problems stem from man's inability to sit quietly in a room alone." - Blaise Pascal, Pensees

It has never been more important to utilise the power of silence. As previously stated, we are all inundated with copious information in the form of technology and marketing that silence is a true blessing. It is our responsibility to reduce the obstacles around us, and increase clarity and deeper thinking. Silence is where flow originates, but this is what people shy away from. If we do not condition ourselves to think positively and calmly in silence, then moments of forced silence (before sleeping,

243

upon waking and when noise is inappropriate) will consist of copious negativity and trepidation. The self grows most in moments of silence. During these moments, the mind may wander, yet we develop the skill to focus on what we want by concentrating and keeping the mind centred. Silence and meditation, in all its forms, harmoniously bring mind and body, and thought and action together. If we are stressed and encounter negative thoughts about relationships and inept areas, then we reduce the ability to pump quality, positive thoughts into our subconscious.

"When you connect to the silence within you, that is when you can make sense of the disturbance going on around you." – Stephen Richards

People who dislike being on their own tend to dislike their inner dialogue. These are the people who would benefit most from sitting in silence with their thoughts, reflecting upon how they think and feel. They can change the negative wiring in their minds by appreciating what they have, focusing more on others and planning a beautiful future for themselves. Think of what you least want to do; this is the thing you need to do most. If you really want to know yourself, simply sit in silence and observe: what do you think about? How do your ideas and visuals interchange? What images come to mind and in what form? What does your inner dialogue encompass? Be very careful about how you communicate with yourself.

Silence is the sound of success. Why are yoga, fasting and exercise so potent? These activities convey just how appreciative and grateful we are to be alive: to breathe, feel and love. We get so absorbed in our lives over futile

244

and nonsensical things: Who has what? Who screwed whom over? How many things do you have? How many friends do you have? How beautiful am I? The three activities mentioned take us away from all of that. The focus shifts onto our basic physiological needs: I am hungry; my heart is thumping; my breathing is so slow; how long can I do this for? What's keeping me alive? So many existential questions come to mind. It takes us back to the basics, so that we can put things into perspective again: nothing is promised to us; we must make the most of our aliveness. We get to focus on things that are so fundamental; things that test us mentally and physically.

Without these therapeutic activities, we lose our ability to take a step back, to view ourselves from the outside, and to consider our true potential. Without them we become infused and consumed with all that is fake and superficial: the ego's pleasures. This is when people become greedy, malevolent and cynical. They become so consumed in competition and material needs, wanting to get one over the other, and to compare themselves with others in what is often a detrimental, unnecessary comparison. We must want to always improve and set high expectations for ourselves without the judgment and involvement of others. Developing the ability to think positively in moments of silence is one of the most important things we can ever master in life. It will improve our discipline, focus and self-esteem. It can certainly positively or negatively affect how we think, feel and act, and it therefore influences our physical shape and overall health.

"Silence is a source of great strength." - Lao Tzu

Accept and Appreciate

"Gratitude unlocks the fullness of life. It turns what we have into enough, and more. It turns denial into acceptance, chaos to order, confusion to clarity." – Melody Beattie

The loving father took his daughter to the ice-cream van. She shouted in joy that she wanted vanilla ice cream, and so the benevolent father got her two scoops of vanilla ice cream on a cone. As they were walking away, she dropped her ice cream on the floor. Uncontrollably, the little girl was moaning that it was heavy, and she lost her grip. Diligently, the father took her back to the van, and asked for one scoop of vanilla ice cream this time, but the child demanded that she wanted three scoops! Intelligently, the father firmly stated, "you could not handle two scoops, so why should we get you three scoops?" Adults can be like this in many ways (and sometimes still about ice-cream). We must love what we have currently manifested in our world, and only then can we come from a place of strength, so that we can handle our 'three scoops' when the time is right. When the student is ready, the teacher will arrive.

We cannot always be in control otherwise we would never experience anew. We would not grow or be flexible enough to react competently and with conviction. When we are grateful for what we have, then we can never be fearful. When people wear flashy things, they communicate less. When people look for a fight, they show true weakness. When people look to dominate others, they push others away. The loudest can is the emptiest. Create the visible by focusing on the invisible. All physical manifestations are a result of how we think, feel and act. When we begin to cultivate true gratefulness, we begin to strip away all of the unnecessary garbage that overwhelm us, enabling us to make better decisions about our health and physical goals. When we come from a place of strength and fullness, we no longer look to take anything and everything (often unhealthy treats) because we already feel abundant, and do not need to scavenge for things that are often unimportant.

Express love and gratefulness to others and yourself. Take a moment to look at yourself in the mirror, and, even though it may sound contradictory, focus on the part of your body that you least like. It could your belly, love handles, chest, bottom or thighs. Anything. Stare at that area, and communicate to yourself that you are exactly the way you are supposed to be at this moment in time. For example, if you do not like your belly, look at it and say the following: "My belly is exactly how it is supposed to be right now. I accept myself in every way." We have been taught to be insecure and dwell on what is wrong with us. When we do this, we cannot focus on the wonderful things about us. I am not advocating that we ignore things that we want to improve, but we must not let these issues define or bother us. Just because we are saying we accept ourselves, it does not mean that we are still not driven to lose fat. It just means we do not need to approach fat loss from this angry, limited perspective.

The same can be done with other things we dislike such as our reactions or ways of thinking about something. For example, if you do not like that you sweat profusely when anxious, then repeat the following: "I appreciate how my body and nervous system reacts when in what appears to be a challenging situation. It shows exactly how I feel, and I accept how I react in these situations. Sweating is natural, and it is a beautiful response that my body chooses, as it does what is natural in this moment." The beauty of such self-accepting and self-loving behaviour is that, ironically, by accepting our flaws, our flaws will fade or dramatically reduce. Why? We give power to what we focus on. When we despise our flaws, we intensify its power (emotion), and we strengthen its response; we ooze hate, and manifest strong emotions that are counterproductive. Conversely, when we love our so-called flaws, we become detached from any self-defeating and limiting thoughts. This opens the possibility for change, and for letting go. We must learn to appease and love ourselves if we are to make healthier choices. We all know what we should and should not eat and drink regularly, yet we often make these mistakes because we cannot control how we communicate with ourselves.

Flexibility

*"Stay committed to your decisions, but stay
flexible in your approach."*
– Tony Robbins

Our physical flexibility represents how flexible and open
we are as people. Rigidity, in the physical form, is a
representation of the mind's inability to simply go with
things. Inflexibility can be linked to stubbornness and
narrow-mindedness. The narrow mind limits experiences
and ways of thinking. If we want to be open minded, and
to feel like we can adapt well to various situations, then
we should physically stretch and become nimble. A body
that flows well, and moves well, is a mind that flows well
and thinks well. The mind and body are incredibly
intertwined. One is always influencing the other. Our
bodies can benefit from physically stretching every single
day.

As it relates to relationships, Tony Robbins exclaims that,
in an interaction, the person who is more certain and
mentally flexible will hold greater control and power.
Why? They have greater resources to draw from. They
have more options open to them. The most flexible
person is the most powerful in any situation as they have
unlimited ways of changing and adapting to be successful
in the interaction. The most versatile person has the most
control. The rigid and stubborn cannot adapt to any
conversation and engage as well with many other people.
The person with the most choices available has the best
chance of choosing one that it most helpful and

supportive. Another analogy can help: the boxer will almost always lose a fight against the mixed martial artist. Why? The boxer is very skilled but one-dimensional whereas the martial artist has an array of attacks that bemuses and staggers the boxer into hesitation and mental chaos. Interestingly, brilliant boxers will actually not be able to box at their potential because they become so overwhelmed due to the opponent's ability to dictate the entire competition. This is how our interactions are with anyone and in any situation! The more physically and mentally open we are, and the more we can flow with things, the more opportunities we have to thrive in live, which will indirectly have an amazing effect on our ability to create the body we want.

Cancel Consistency

Understandably, I know why you might initially interpret this as ironic (because I have been expressing the need for consistency and congruency in our thoughts, emotions and behaviours). However, we cannot be consistent with the way we have been so far in our lives if we are to make massive positive changes to our health and bodies. Instead, we must change our thoughts, emotions and actions. We must literally become a new version of ourselves (like installing the latest version on our phone's settings) by reflecting on what has worked up until now, and what has not worked for us up until now. We must change who we are. We must change our personality. Our bodies constantly change its cells, and so, in terms of our cellular structure, we are literally new people every several years. If this is the case, why might it seem unusual to want to change who we are? This is what growth actually means: becoming a better version of what you once were, and thus cannot be accomplished with the same thoughts, emotions and actions that have currently got us where we are. We must instil powerful, supportive habits first, and then we must become consistent with these newly installed habits. We have to rewire our brains otherwise we will keep getting the results we have got until now. Consider the thoughts, emotions and actions you do every single day. What ones would you like to replace? What would you like to replace them with? We must therefore condition ourselves to override our current negativity by immediately firing positive statements until these positive reactions become automatic.

Take Action

***"An idea not coupled with action will never get any bigger than the brain cell it occupied."* - Arnold Glasow**

Bring certainty to the uncertainty otherwise uncertainty will pervade what was once a certainty! Have you ever worked for someone with whom you thought you were more skilled and talented than? Obviously there are different variables: experience, luck, gender and so forth. However, if there were not these variables, why is that person more successful financially than you in terms of your occupation? It is most likely these two things: likeability and taking action. Stop talking about what you need to do, and just do what you need to do. Just make a start. You will notice that you talk less this way, and actually accomplish more. The thought of taking action deters many. It is the fear of the unknown; it is the fear of change; it is the fear of not being in control. Yes, it is imperative to think things through rather than leaping into danger ignorantly, yet there is a great deal of pain and resentfulness built over time by people who do not take action for what they need or want for themselves and their future. Unfortunately, they tend to blame others rather than take responsibility for their current circumstance. Know what actions you need to take each day, and block out a certain amount of time to carry out each of these essentials such as exercising, meditating, planning your meals and eating these meals.

Inopportunely, many people simply do not take action because they feel they are unequipped with the necessary skills to take the plunge. They fear that they will feel judged, criticised and disparaged if they make a mistake or fail. Failure is the only way to achieve success. To fail means we took a step forward. Coming up short is a sign that we must improve, so that we become more adept and successful. How will we find this out unless we go for it? Why did I write this book? There are many more ideas and information I could have read, learned, incorporated, expanded upon and deciphered, but many works are left unfinished because of this obsession to make things perfect (which is of course unattainable). But I wrote. I put pen to paper, and I hope you are able to do your best, and just produce the best that you can. What things do you not partake in because you are concerned that you will not execute them outstandingly? Write a list. What factors cause you to restrain from taking part? Are you concerned that it will not amount to anything? Are you concerned about what others will think? Are you concerned that you may not be as good as you thought (a downfall of following the ego again)? We must overcome this mental hurdle that burdens us, and that affects our emotions, which indirectly affects how we choose to eat and exercise.

Self-Reflection

"The unexamined life is not worth living." - Socrates

We want to build our metaphorical house (our bodies) by looking at it from the outside rather than the inside. If we are inside when building, then it is harder to see the problems and issues within the house, as we are too close to the experience. We must step back, build gradually, and step back frequently in order to preempt any issues, so that we can design it impeccably. The best in every field are those who are constantly stepping back, and returning to their work with new insight and perspectives. This requires a great deal of objectivity and detachment from the ego. Many people cannot be completely honest with themselves because they immerse themselves in their egos. We must work incredibly hard in areas that we deem to be important to us (such as our health and physical goals), and we will become successful and satisfied in that avenue. However, the ability to step back and evaluate ourselves is fundamental. This is when we reassess, and make small adjustments to keep us on track most efficiently and effectively.

Living a life dominated by our egos is very painful. Our fall becomes that much more tragic and brutal. We all experience similar thoughts and emotions throughout our lives, yet there are some people who take action in spite of what is going on inside. Once we take action, our challenging thoughts and feelings about whatever is happening will change because we have newer references and experiences. Nature and fate will take its course if we do not take action, and we will encounter greater pain consequentially. The seemingly negative and painful things that happen to us, end up being the most substantial, essential and transformational events. However, we need to condition our reactions to what has happened; otherwise we can allow these events to get the better of us. We can either use our perceived failures to make us better, or we can allow them to break us. When someone fails at something, they do one of two things: despondent individuals will associate themselves, and define themselves by this result: "I failed," "I am a loser," "I am not good enough," "This is who I am," and this downtrodden person will visualise a lack of success every time they encounter similar situations, further associating themselves with failing visually; resilient, detached individuals react differently, saying things such as, "Oh it didn't work out this time," "I am going to come back stronger," "I am better than that," "This loss will only make me better," "I am more than this outcome." It is in our struggles and challenges where we learn most about who we are. When we win, we celebrate; when we lose, we contemplate. Therefore, we learn and grow more when we 'lose' or 'fail.' The faster we 'fail,' the more quickly we will succeed. Fail intelligently.

Become Detached

"Detachment is not that you should own nothing. But that nothing should own you." Ali ibn abi Talib

We must turn all the negative feelings we have, especially if they relate to food, into pure thoughts. We want to make decisions based on our thoughts rather than our emotions. People usually buy things based on emotions, and they justify them with logic, but if we are to do what is best for ourselves, then we must do the opposite: make decisions based on logic, and use our powerful emotions to drive this logic forward. Get into the habit of asking yourself these questions before you eat every meal: Will this support me? Is this good for me? Will eating this make me weaker or stronger? As with all habits, they take time until they become fully embedded, so be patient and persistent. There will be times when this will become annoying and perhaps even tedious, but the juice is worth the squeeze. Just think of all the heartache and struggle you will avoid by constantly questioning what you are about to eat and why.

It may seem like hyperbole, but if you do not own your relationship with food, then food will end up owning you. Read the following sentence: "Emma ate the cake." The object, the cake, is not the enemy; food is not the enemy. It is our internal processes, and our stress, that is the enemy. Therefore, 'Emma' must take responsibility because she is the only one who can experience thoughts and emotions in this statement. Unhealthy or healthy eating has nothing to do with the food itself; it is all about what is happening within us that result in this unhealthy eating. Food itself is not the enemy; our stress is the enemy. Our stress induces our thought, emotions and actions, and so really, our personality is determined by how we react to different forms of stress (physical and mental). Stress is everywhere, and so we cannot ever get rid of stress completely, but we can determine how we react to it.

Let us analyse the processes involved when we eat unhealthy foods. The most significant moment is not what happens when we are actually eating the unhealthy foods; it is what happens before we begin to eat. It is more about the thoughts and emotions we experience, or do not experience, leading up to our unhelpful choices. What are the reasons for eating unhealthily? Is it because we have not eaten much, and so we eat voraciously and often foods that we know will 'get the job done?' Is it because we feel stressed out, and we know we are about to do something that we do not really want to do (write an email, go into that boring meeting, begin that new project etc.), and so it is a way of calming ourselves down? Is it because everyone is gathering to eat or snack, and everything on display is unhealthy, and thus we want to fit in? Moreover, some people just want to do and not think. They simply eat, and do not even take the time to contemplate eating. Unfortunately, this is probably even more damaging. Why? They are clearly not investing time and energy into contemplating whether or not they should be eating something. They simply begin eating whatever they feel like eating. Just as previously mentioned, many people buy with emotions and justify with logic, and this is the exact same thing that people do when deciding what to eat: they eat based on emotions, and they justify why they ate like that after (in order to appease themselves, and prove that they were right to do it).

What actual events take place before you usually eat unhealthily? Have you just finished working for a few hours and it is your break? Did you just have an argument with someone? Did you just have a workout, and so you think it is not as harmful to eat what you want after? Once you know what events lead to this unsupportive habit, the next step is to write down all of the feelings you have before you eat like this; we must then uncover what you experience after eating this food. For example, hunger creates a form of physical stress, and so eating is a way of calming ourselves down, so that we can focus on other priorities. Mental stress is a form of fear, and so we may eat unhealthily to make us forget, momentarily, about what we are experiencing or what we were recently experiencing. It is an emotional distraction. Wanting to fit in is also a form of fear, as we do not wish to be cast aside and boycotted, and so eating unhealthily with others can make us feel connected and therefore accepted.

Once we explicitly know what is happening and why, then we can choose better options. We can become more proactive, and plan our day better (choosing an earlier time to eat or drink something for example), so that we do not have to eat ravenously. We can preempt that we will feel more stressed out at certain times in the day (before meetings, making a certain phone call, deadline day etc.), and so we can embed robust affirmations and stress-relieving routines either in the morning or preceding these more challenging moments (these will be shared in chapter 10). Moreover, we can directly tell others what our goals are (eating healthily), and still enjoy the company of our peers without having to indulge in their naughty festivities.

We want to cut off all emotions attached when eating unhealthy foods. Do you eat unhealthily because you are feeing sorry for yourself (victim mentality)? Is it because you want to fit in with a peer group (out of fear)? Is it because you feel overwhelmed and need a quick release (poor emotional intelligence)? Instead we must develop powerful emotions when we see or think of healthier alternatives. We must condition ourselves to love seeing salads, vegetables and healthy foods because we know how good they are for us. We know that they support our minds and bodies. Also, we want to condition ourselves to conjure negative associations to unhealthy foods that will add fat to our bodies. Listen to the following foods, and write down the first emotion or idea that comes to mind. Are you ready? 1) Triple chocolate-layered cake. 2) Salad. 3) Kebab. 4) Salmon. You may find it useful to write emotive adjectives to describe these foods in ways that will support future decision-making. For example, disease-inducing triple chocolate-layered cake; superfood rainbow salad; disgusting artery-clogging kebab, and delicious salmon. The words we use condition how we feel about the foods. Moreover, the way we visualise these foods in our minds (when they are and when they are not in front of us) will either put us off or want the foods even more. Imagine all the nasty fatty oil dripping off the kebab and what that will do to your insides. Conversely, imagine the beautifully colourful, fresh salad revitalising your taste buds, and how light and energetic it will make you feel after.

The Passenger

Arguably the most important thing to do for our health and physical goals is to live our lives as though we are in the passenger's seat of the 'car.' The more detached we can be from what we are experiencing, the easier it is to make the correct choices. Have you ever sat in the passenger's seat, and felt different to the person who was actually driving the car? Have you noticed how the actual driver tends to be more emotional, and tends to take things personally when driving and interacting with other drivers? Have you also noticed how the passenger invariably seems calmer and less agitated when other drivers, or things, exhibit negative and disrespectful behaviour?

We must live our lives as though we are passengers. Why? We will make fewer mistakes because we will be less emotionally engaged, and thus more logical, in all that is happening around us. We will be able to physically and metaphorically see more in terms of the overall picture because we are more focused on the journey than the mechanics of what is happening. We are more likely to experience flow because flow can be experienced more readily when the conscious mind is less involved. Take control of your life by omnisciently and objectively perceiving everything that unfolds inside and outside of our experience.

The more emotional we are, the more docile we are. If things (products or services) are bought based on emotion, then emotional people are susceptible to being influenced more easily. If we are always immersed in our experiences, then we are more emotional, and thus more likely to be swayed by external factors: the alluring smell of junk food as we walk down the high-street; our friends randomly deciding to go for dinner and everyone therefore orders unhealthy food and drink. If we are emotional, then we experience joy, excitement, anxiety and fear more readily. This means that we can change very quickly: we can go from being in control and content one moment to being angry and thus wanting to change our state quickly through food etc. If we want to live more healthily, then we must either become less emotional generally or develop our emotional intelligence: being able to control our emotions and how we feel, so that we can make better choices more often.

Chapter 9: Mechanics - Keep Active and Busy

Interestingly, much of our physical success happens when we are not exercising or eating. It is in the moments in between. One of the main ways that we can ensure we remain on the healthy path is to keep ourselves motivated, active and busy. We need to cultivate a more enjoyable and exciting life in general if we are to consistently and easily make the right choices. It does not matter who we are, if we are frequently bored, frustrated or stressed, then we will make poorer decisions more often. We must consider how we spend much of our day, and how this affects our responses in relation to eating and exercising.

Boredom and Inertia

"Boredom: the desire for desires." – Leo Tolstoy

We should seldom experience boredom in our lives. There is so much to learn, do and create. Boredom often results from ineffectively planning our day, weeks, months and even years. Boredom is experienced more by those who are more reactive, and, therefore, less proactive. Personally, I only ever experience boredom sometimes in between meetings for a few minutes, and only if I forgot to bring a notepad or paper, otherwise I would be planning or creating something. Boredom leads to negative thinking, which leads to us needing instant gratification, which oftentimes leads to eating unhealthily. We must live such a fulfilling, active and captivating life, that we simply do not think about food or drinks, especially the bad ones, that often. It should rarely cross our minds. The more mediocre our lives feel, the more we feel the need to fill this missing hole, and this is most lazily done by eating more and worse foods. These poor eating choices, then end up making us feel more sluggish and lethargic, which again takes away even more energy from us, ensuring that we do not do more empowering things with our times such as starting a business or exploring new things or taking our hobbies to the highest levels and so on. This is a perilous cycle that drags us deeper into quick sand.

Inertia is a prerequisite for depression. It is the middle ground between sadness and depression. We must create a lifestyle where our mind and/or bodies are being put to good use. Boredom should not even take place when we are tired. Exhaustion can sometimes occur as a consequence of doing too much especially taxing things where we require great focus. However, even when we rest, we do not feel bored. Boredom occurs when we have some energy at least, yet we do not know what to do with it. We must feel that something must change whenever we feel bored. There is so much to do and experience in this world that we should never experience boredom. This is a great opportunity for us to plan our lives better now. What would inspire us more? What would keep us busier? What would make us more fulfilled? Do we need to get a different partner? Do we need more holidays? Do we need a new career? Do we need to live in a better area? Do we need to put our money to better use? There is a closer connection between our careers and our relationship with food than we think.

Usually people overeat and over think when they are bored or feel lonely, and have nothing meaningful to do. This is a result of the long-term thinking and emotional patterns that have accumulated over years. It is the result of poor quality decisions for a sustained period of time. Fortunately, this can be changed in an instant. We must just decide to change it. We must understand where we have gone wrong in the past, and then we must literally create a new personality (new thoughts about ourselves, the world and people, and new emotions that inspire and excite). Conversely, overtraining and being too physically active can result in overeating as well. We might feel so sore, stiff and shattered that we feel like we need to consume so much more in order to recover and recuperate. Balance is necessary. Moreover, even if we trained for several hours every day, then we are more likely not putting enough energy and effort into other important things such as creating a more captivating and exciting lifestyle. What good is it training for several hours in the day if we are working a job that brings us no real joy and not enough finances to reduce our stress levels? Things are all connected. We want to avoid both extremes: we must avoid boredom by planning and being active mentally and physically, yet we need to know when we are pushing ourselves mentally and physically too hard. This comes down to discipline, and providing quality time every day for each important aspect in our lives: health, wealth and relationships.

Distractions

"Nothing lasts forever – not even your troubles."
– Arnold H. Glasow

We must understand that feelings and sensations come and go. Many people think that the way things are now is the way they will be for a long time. This belief exists across many different areas in life, but it also exists when it comes to our states. What comes to us now, will leave us soon and vice versa. There will be times when we feel unusually hungry, or when we are more susceptible to eating junk food. Understand that this moment will pass and often very soon. It is all about doing whatever we can to avoid giving in during those very brief moments (often lasting seconds or a few minutes). We must choose and embed strategies that we can call upon during these moments. It might be useful to cultivate an experience of flow: partaking in an activity that requires our absolute focus. This will result in us forgetting about the sensations we had previously. This is not one of my favourite strategies, but it is effective if we even partake in a stressful activity, as stress, at times, can make us lose our appetite; we become so focused on an activity, in this instance a stressful one (such as responding to an urgent email or completing an urgent task), that we completely forget that our stomachs were just growling or that we were thinking about what unhealthy foods we could be eating and so on.

We must develop affirmations and incantations to override the negative voice that wants us to give in, or we can simply remind ourselves of our goals, and why we want to achieve them. This will keep us focused. We know that excuses are for the weak. We must believe that otherwise we will be able to justify our unhealthy eating. That would be a recipe for disaster. If we teach ourselves that eating unhealthily is for the weak, then we will presume that we are weak if we give in. This is not something that most healthy people want to think and feel about themselves. Therefore, it is a great strategy. People who think that these associations (weakness because of eating decisions) are unfair or unjust tend to be the very people who are unhealthy and overweight. If we are overweight or not where we want to be, then we must know how to trigger ourselves. We must know how to attack our own egos, so that we make better choices for our health and physical shape. For example, I wake myself up at five in the morning every single day, regardless of when I went to sleep. As you can imagine, sometimes I do not want to get out of bed at that time. I therefore communicate with myself in a way that musters enough intensity and emotion that I get out of bed and begin doing the productive things I do every single morning. I might think something like, "You are a quitter if you do not get up now," or "What would (insert role model's name) do if he/she was in my position right now?" Understand how to motivate yourself, and do it whenever you need that extra push!

We can preempt or mitigate these vulnerable moments depending on how well we know ourselves, and what kind of day, or few hours, we know we are going to have.

Again, this is where our emotional intelligence can support us further. For example, if we know that we have a long and stressful meeting the following day, then we can anticipate that we will be mentally or emotionally weaker before and/or soon after the meeting. If we know how we operate, then we can be prepared. Do we usually like to calm ourselves down before such meetings (usually in the form of food), or are we more likely to eat unhealthily after the meeting as a way of rewarding ourselves for enduring the meeting? We can proactively presume our emotional state during certain moments, and thus be ready for these states and emotions: "That meeting was just as tough as I thought it would be. I know I feel like treating myself, but this is the wrong move. I am going to just stay calm and rest instead." If your emotions are very strong at this time, then you can deliver an incantation, such as, "I will remain on track because I am stronger than any external event." It is better to plan stress-reducing activities before and after such events, so that we appease ourselves in the best ways possible. This can be by meditating or exercising in the morning to relieve that tension, or by scheduling a nice walk in the park for after the event and so forth.

Reduce Stress

"Adopting the right attitude can convert a negative stress into a positive one." – Hans Selye

Stress can be defined as a form of tension or pressure. It is oftentimes a build up of anxiety, and, thus, it is a negative feeling that can be linked to fear. All people have conditioned themselves to deal with stress in their own ways. Stress occurs when we feel overwhelmed. We must detach ourselves from these feelings of stress (fear) by mentally and physically stepping back from what we are experiencing. We must put our stress into context and into perspective by considering what really matters to us, and what we should be grateful for: breathing, being able to spend time with our loved ones, having somewhere to stay and sleep. When we return to the most basic needs during moments of stress, then we can appease ourselves, and return to these challenging tasks with greater clarity and peace.

Firstly, hear are some examples of unhealthy ways people deal with stress: illicit drugs; alcohol; argumentation; fighting; bullying others (more frequent that you may think among adults); delegation without providing necessary support; masochistic activities and so on. Here are some more supportive ways people can release stress: going for long walks; meditation/yoga; exercise; playing sport; reading; listening to music; being alone; being with loved ones; seeing friends; cleaning or fixing things; flow inducing activities and so on. Consider the ways in which you reduce stress, and if this short-term stress reducer carries any long-term stress. Smoking, for example, can reduce stress and our appetite. However, in the long term, smoking will obviously lead to awful side effects and potential illnesses that carry even greater stress or worse. Write down the short-term effects of your stress-reducing choices, and then write down any long-term effects they may have.

Stress is not actually the biggest problem. In many ways, it is rather challenging to not experience stress because we obviously feel that we must get a lot done within a short period of time. It is understandable that we feel stress because of this. However, it is important to consider who has created this stress, and if it is necessary. Are you making yourself stressed because of unrealistic expectations of what you can accomplish during a short period of time? Are you stressed because of the pressure a loved one is putting you under? Are you stressed because of your employer or line manager setting extremely challenging tasks with short deadlines? You can change all three situations. You have a choice. For example, maybe you are the one who needs to put things into perspective, and to have more realistic expectations of what can be achieved within a day or week. If a loved one is unnecessarily stressing you, then either spend less time with this person, have conversations with them about how they are making you feel, or choose to not have this person as part of your life anymore. If an employer or line manager puts you under great stress, and often, then simply find a new job, become self-employed or start a new business. It is that simple. No one should be made to feel overly stressed by anyone especially consistently. This must be one of your life principles.

Flow

"Flow is being completely involved in an activity for its own sake. The ego falls away. Time flies. Every action, movement, and thought follows inevitably from the previous one, like playing jazz."
– Mihaly Csikszentmihalyi

If we are to develop the kind of lifestyle that will enable us to live happily and make smarter decisions for our bodies, then we must increase the intensity and amount of times we experience flow on a daily basis. Firstly, please read, *Flow* by Mihaly Csikszentmihalyi, as it brilliantly breaks down the constituents that enable the state known as flow. Let us explore the diverse elements that must occur for us to experience flow, and, thus, enjoy things to the maximum (not only significant activities such as creating, performing and presenting).

Experiencing flow occurs when we are so immersed in what we are doing that nothing else matters or disturbs our thought. This hyperbolic phrase emphasises the type of focus, drive and clarity necessary to achieve flow. In these moments, we do not allow any intrusions to deter our thoughts, feelings and actions. We are so in tune with the present moment that we are unable to question ourselves. During this experience, it is common for people to view themselves from outside of the box, and to think of the bigger picture, our roles in this universe, who feels our energy vibrations and how this might this transcend into other people's relationships. When people

271

are performing at their best, and when they are experiencing flow, they explain the experience as though it is not them who is doing it. They feel as though they are watching themselves, almost like they are playing a computer game.

The less you think, the better you perform.

The subconscious is in full swing whenever we experience a state of flow. Our conscious can often get in the way even though it is only trying to protect us sometimes. If we master a skill, then whenever we perform this skill, we will want to remove our conscious thinking as much as possible. The removal of our conscious thoughts will enable flow. During flow, there is no thought; there is only fluid action and trust. To experience flow we must be so competent and focused on something that we enter a positive trance. We enter a hypnotic state when we experience flow. This is when the subconscious is allowed to run the show, and our habitual skills are capable of flourishing. We lose this extraordinary experience when we begin thinking about what we are doing.

Internal talk must cease. Even positive self-talk does not help as much when wanting to access flow. Any hesitation of thought, and the moment of magic becomes lost in translation. A frail, older woman was able to lift a car to save her child who was caught under the wheel. How? There was no thought. Her subconscious took control in its most instinctive way. If there was a moment where her conscious intervened and took hold of this circumstance, then that child may not have survived. If for a moment she thought, "There's no way I can lift this car," or "I cannot save my son," then she would have fatally faltered. Pure love and focus dictated action and belief. She refused to allow any externality to prevent such heroism. In moments of success, we do not need to think; we do not need to *try* or force anything. We just allow ourselves to let go, because we trust ourselves enough to let go in these moments, and we will naturally know what to say or how to move. To experience flow, we cannot think things through; we must simply allow the mind and body to do what come naturally.

Flow is all about achieving the perfect harmony between our subconscious mind and body. If our mind is truly relaxed, totally clear, then we will achieve flow more easily. This is why yoga, mediation, and conditioning the mind to be free of thought, or close to no thought, will result in operating fluidly and smoothly. It is like driving a car on a bumpy road: we can never really relax if we have to be aware of all of the bumps in the road. These bumps are our thoughts intruding upon our mental clarity, and, thus, our ability to access flow. Every thought and action flows interchangeably. There is no room for doubt or hesitation if we want to access our best state: flow. The more we simplify our lives, the more mental clarity we have, and the more clarity and peace we have, the more readily we can access flow. Flow-inducing activities must be appropriately challenging in order to demand complete focus. It must not be overly familiar (too easy), and it must not be overly novel (too hard). This is why we must build up the level of complexity and challenge gradually, so that we stay within flow.

In order to access flow, we must be able to hypnotise ourselves. We are still aware of things, but it is the difference between being the person who is playing the computer game (being detached and in flow), or being the character in the game (too close to the action and unable to experience flow as thoughts and emotions intrude too much). Think and do as you would when feeling these positive and empowering states. We are most confident when we feel like we can be ourselves. Utmost confidence is displayed when people experience flow, as they do not allow any hesitation or self-consciousness to disenable their aptitude. We can relax, and literally allow the actions to unfold in front of us. We must do what feels natural to us in that moment. The more we experience flow, the less likely we are to eat unhealthily and emotionally. We will cultivate so much natural energy and joy from being immersed in interesting activities that we will eat better. This is why it is so important to love what you do for a living because it will massively help you with your body shape. Contemplate the things that you do weekly, if not daily, that enable you to access flow. See if you can do this more often, so that we create amazing states and energy. This will do wonders for our decision-making as it relates to our health and bodies. Additionally, consider some of the things that you currently do that can be changed, so that you are more likely to experience flow and appropriate stimulation. Conversely, think about the things you do daily that are not pleasurable. See if you can eliminate these where possible as low energy vibrations will result in the need for more external stimulation (oftentimes in the form of unhealthy foods).

Our Purpose

"Choose your friends with caution; plan your future with purpose, and frame your life with faith." – Thomas S. Monson

Find your purpose. Have big goals. Set high standards in significant areas. Make time for your purpose and priorities every single day. When you feel like you are progressing at something meaningful, then you become immersed in the experience, and you will not feel the need to eat as a distraction. Instead, you will not want distractions! You will simply view eating food as adding fuel, so that you can focus more on your purpose and priorities. There is a monumental difference between these perceptions. We want to become so absorbed in what we do for a living that we do not even contemplate that we have not eaten anything for a long time. We want to have forgotten that we skipped a meal rather than watching the clock all the time thinking about when we will next eat.

If our purpose is compelling enough, then everything else should fall into place. If our purpose is so important in influencing our shape, then what happens if we do not know our purpose yet? Everyone has a purpose. If we have not found ours yet, then we are not exploring enough. We have not yet challenged ourselves in enough avenues to tie our strengths together into a singular focus. For example, I know my purpose was to help people to achieve their goals, dreams and potential: I have a deep love for psychology and philosophy; I love to keep physically and mentally strong and healthy. It was only natural for me to express my ideas and experiences in these kind of platforms. My strengths came together, and I naturally fell into this career because I was always researching and experimenting with new things. Consider where you are currently, and if it is your idyllic purpose. If not, then write down your current strengths, and then write your current interests. Then see how you can tie as many of these together, and research what kind of professions they fall into. Simply experience different professions or avenues until one just feels right for you. Then master this skill, and enjoy the flow-inducing challenges that await you.

For us to remain inspired and transfixed in our purpose, we must constantly look to improve, so that we continue to affect more people and in even more meaningful ways. Plan out your journey for the next five to ten years: what do you want to achieve by then and by when? What will you need to achieve first? What about in five years from now? Once we know these things, then we should write down the actions we must complete in order to achieve these goals one-step at a time. If we are genuinely very happy with these goals, and its order, then we must strictly adhere to this plan. You may become tempted to avoid certain steps or change things, but resist this urge if you are happy with the long-term plan. Remain focused on this path no matter what obstacles or problems show up.

Our purpose and physical shape are very closely tied together. The more lost we feel in our careers, the more we will require short-term gratification in order to get us through the daily grind. People who know their purpose also tend to work extremely hard as well, but in ways that support their self-esteem. People on their purpose feel greater pleasure in what they do, and so they have the inner strength and energy to fight stronger in other areas. If people see their jobs as a fight that they must survive every day, then they will not be able to fight well in other areas of life, which include our health and physical shape. If our careers enable us to experience flow, excitement and possibility every day, then we have the inner peace and pleasure within to show up strong in other areas. It is the equivalent of sending two soldiers to war for the same mission (staying healthy and in physical shape for instance); one soldier is rested and robust whereas the other has been deeply wounded. The same applies to us, and what we experience. The more mental and emotional wounds we deal with each day, the less strength we have to surmount other challenges such as our health and wellbeing.

Having a career that excites us enables us to make better choices throughout the day. We will be able to deal with obstacles better if we feel like we are on our journey, and that we are doing well. This massively affects our mindset as it relates to eating healthily and training well. It is all about momentum and discipline. Our discipline in one area can infiltrate other areas. Think about what makes you good at your profession, and see how many of these tasks or skills you can transfer to your health and body-shape goals. The more commonalities we can find between the different disciplines in our lives (health, relationships and wealth), then the easier it is to integrate these skills and routines together. This is metacognition:

knowing how we learn and when we are at our best, and linking these together in important areas, so that we consistently follow certain procedures successfully. Keep doing what works!

Mind Games

"Chances are you're using overeating as a way to escape yourself. It's an attempt not to feel or think about what you really need to feel and face."
- Karen Salmansohn

We will constantly fight against our emotions as it relates to food unless we change our perceptions. Unfortunately, some people do not attack the root cause of the problem (their associations and perceptions around food and drink). Instead, they go on diets where they try to use willpower alone to surmount their urges. This will only last for a short period of time, and usually the rebound effect is even worse: people end up eventually gaining more fat than they had before they went on the diet! They set themselves up for failure because they have not rewired their minds; they are using the same faulty mental and emotional connections in order to achieve something different. This is the definition of insanity! It does not matter how mentally tough we are, life will always batter toughness alone. We need the right psychology not the right toughness because we can never fight forever. We must learn to dance with our beliefs, associations and thoughts. They will not always serve us, and so we must appease ourselves and motivate ourselves consistently.

If we are struggling to change our perceptions around food and drink, then there is another way to utilise will power better, however, this is probably unsustainable. We must have continuous short-term physical goals in order to keep us on the right track. People who have one short-term physical goal, such as getting into shape for their forthcoming holiday, will do very well up until the event, but then they will totally let themselves go after the holiday. This takes them back to square one. People who do this are usually short-term thinkers, and so they will always struggle with their body-shape goals. If you know you are like this, then you can beat your own mental processes by constantly coming up with short-term exciting goals to keep you motivated enough to defeat your emotional impulses. For example, let us look at a yearly plan of small goals to keep an individual like this on track:

January: New Year's Resolution to lose five pounds
February: Birthday weekend
March: Susan's wedding
April: Spring-break parties
May: Holiday in Turkey
June: Sessions with a personal trainer
July: High School reunion
August: Holiday in Las Vegas
September: Annual health check up
October: Halloween party
November: Meeting or seeing old acquaintances
December: New Year's Party

Have a new event set up for each month, so that you remain excited and motivated. This is easier for extroverts as they tend to be invited to more parties etc. We do not want to treat eating as an experience unless we are at a party or a celebration. Eating should only be viewed as an opportunity to fuel our minds and bodies. It is one of the few times we should not look to experience flow (unless making and eating healthy meals of course!). The more we enjoy eating, and make eating a drawn out activity, the more we will want to eat this way. Take the emotion out of eating.

We must understand that a diet is a short-term solution. Eliminate the noun 'Diet' from your vocabulary. Supplant it with the term, lifestyle. Healthy eating is now a way of life for us. We must eat healthily at least 90% of the time every single week. We must condition our brains to accept that this is a permanent change. It is the way things will be from now on. We need this change to be a must, and not a should! If something is a should, then it means that we are allowing ourselves to go off the path. We always manage to complete things that are musts as they are our priorities. These are things that are not up for negotiation. The more we break these musts, the more we lose trust in ourselves. The more we distrust ourselves, the lower our self-esteem becomes. Our feelings of self-worth will ascertain whether we should stay on the right path or sabotage our own success.

The Easiest Way

"Always do your best. What you plant now, you will harvest later."
– Og Mandino

Small things turn into big things. If we want to always do the most convenient things or wear the most comfortable clothes, then we begin to condition the brain to always look for, and choose, the easiest options or the things that are most comfortable. This may seem smart, but the problem is these small-scale decisions begin to permeate into our core beliefs: "Why should I wake up early to train? I want to be comfortable." "What is the point in joining that Pilates class? It is easier to stay in bed." "Why should I buy that book about health when I know I won't read it?" The easiest way in life can sometimes be the best option, but only once certain contextual factors have been included within its decision-making. For example, is it necessary for me to park as close to the store as possible? Well I have to carry these really heavy things to the car. In this case, the easiest option is the right thing to undertake. Should I go to that one-hour class when I know I have promised to take my friend to gym later in the afternoon? Well I have other things to do today as well, and I will already be training in the afternoon, so it is fine for me to miss the gym class today. These are legitimate reasons to take the easiest option, but be careful because the brain looks to keep us safe, at all times, and thus sabotage our success: the brain will come up with excuses every single time in order to put us off, and unhelpfully this sounds like the exact same voice that gave us legitimate reasons to take the easiest option beforehand.

Unfortunately, there will be times when we choose the easiest options when they should not be taken: "I am not going to go to the gym today because it is Friday, and I have the whole weekend to catch up with training." Wrong attitude! "It is my cheat meal tomorrow, so what is the harm in having something a little naughty just a few hours earlier as well?" Wrong attitude! "Listen I am with my friends, and we are all having a great time, I am going to order whatever suits the situation." Wrong attitude! We must take responsibility, and we must be emotionally intelligent. We must judiciously decide when to listen to that protective voice and when to calm it down and do the right thing even if it is not the easiest option. How can we condition ourselves to choose the best option and not the easiest? Get used to making yourself uncomfortable! We do not have to work hard in order to do what is comfortable as the easiest option is always the first option that comes to mind. We must challenge ourselves. We must evaluate the different options available, and choose the option that best serves our priorities at the time, and our health and physical shape should always be one of our main priorities! Write a list of many decisions that you make every day regarding your physical activities. How many of these decisions are chosen because they are the easiest decisions? How could these be changed if your priority was fat loss and muscle development? Put as many of these into action as of now!

Chapter 10: Mechanics – Routines

"Think in the morning. Act in the noon. Eat in the evening. Sleep in the night." – William Blake

We have conditioned ourselves into performing certain patterns every single day. A routine is the daily execution of the same, or similar, thoughts, emotions and actions. The more often we use these sequences, the stronger they become embedded within our subconscious. They become easier and more effortless to perform. Every single routine becomes easier to perform the more frequently we do them, regardless if it was once a very challenging task. As we become older, it becomes even more challenging to change our routines and habits because we are too fixed and rigid in our beliefs: we have stopped changing our personalities; we have become too good at current routines, and fear the idea of losing our certainty by changing them or adding new ones. This is highly problematic especially if we want to change our minds and bodies. This is also why we must be so driven, determined and disciplined to ensure that we do these newly learned sequences (thought, emotion, action) consistently until we finally create a new pattern.

The most important aspects by far when it comes to our body shape and health is how disciplined we are. Discipline and focus are both important, yet they are quite different. Someone can be focused, but still be inefficient with their time. We can be focused on losing fat and becoming leaner, yet be wasteful with our time and what we accomplish. However, discipline requires that we not only partake in certain activities at certain times each day, but it ensures that we maximise what we produce because of the high standards we have enforced to maintain this discipline. The main characteristic needed to succeed in life and with our bodies is to consistently show up. Show up with the right attitude, regardless of how you feel, and wonderful things will happen. Unfortunately, many people think things like, "I know it's a routine for me to train in the mornings before work, but I know that I will not have a good workout today if I go." That does not matter! It is not always about how well you train at the gym for example. It is more important to just turn up at the gym because that is your promise to yourself. Interestingly, you invariably end up training better than you thought once you warm up and take pressure off yourself to train well. The best in the world, in any field, are not those who do remarkable things necessarily. They just demand that they do things every single day to take themselves closer to their goals. That is all we need to do. Let us explore the many daily physical and mental routines that can profoundly affect our fat-loss and muscle-development goals.

Plan your Day

"Plan your work for today and every day, then work your plan."
— Margaret Thatcher

What is your average day usually like? What activities do you do daily? How much time is roughly allocated to these activities? What times do you wake and go to sleep? What routines do you follow? When do you eat during the day? What do you find time for most days? The more we can accurately plan every hour of our day, the more control we feel regarding our health. We develop consistency when we do the things we know we need to do. We develop consistency when we know we deliver on certain routines every day. It develops trust, self-esteem and ensures that we eat and exercise as we planned. The more control we have, the more discipline we can enforce. The more disciplined we are, the more we can accomplish. The more we accomplish, the greater the momentum we generate. The more momentum we generate, the stronger our self-esteem and positive beliefs become. The stronger our self-esteem, the more careful we are about what we put into our bodies, how we feel and thus how we perform things daily. The entire process continues again and again. It is the success cycle.

If we know what we must accomplish during a given day, then it keeps us on the right path. We avoid doing things randomly (self-sabotaging and procrastination); we avoid getting distracted by pleasant yet long-lasting and meaningless conversations with others with whom we did not plan on meeting; we evade taking on tasks that are unnecessary because we have already prioritised what our work for that given day must be. This not only indirectly affects our health and body, but the same level of focus and discipline directly applies to our eating and training: if we know what we must eat today, and what we must do in the gym, then there is not enough 'room' to meander and partake in unhelpful eating and unhelpful habits. If we all dedicate a certain amount of time, energy and effort into what we eat and our physical movements per day, then once we train and eat the way we intended, there is not much time or energy to get involved with unhealthy meals or going out for drinks. This tends to work more subconsciously. We got our health 'fix,' and so we do not feel the urge to do something random as much.

A similar example is if we force ourselves to wake up early (say five o'clock every morning), then we simply will not have much energy say after eleven o'clock at night, which keeps us more focused, and we subconsciously begin to prioritise the great work and habits instilled in the morning rather than allowing ourselves to capriciously become involved in naughty nighttime antics. Consider the time, energy and effort you allocate to certain habits each day, and see how you can mentally play chess against yourself by instilling certain maneuvers, so that the opponent (yourself) cannot get their decadent way (in the form of negative eating and unsupportive lifestyle habits). Checkmate.

Daily Routines

"The secret of your future is hidden in your daily routine."
– Mike Murdock

We empower ourselves by incorporating uplifting and inspirational daily routines. Consider your daily schedule. Which of these habits drain you, and which of these, even though it requires energy, actually increases energy and enthusiasm? Establish supportive morning and bedtime routines as it will make you feel more in control of your thoughts, emotions and actions throughout the day. Look to supplant your more unhelpful habits with those that add to the quality of your life. Start and finish the day in control. Begin the day with momentum. Please read, *Miracle Morning* by Hal Elrod. Each day should begin with a morning routine. Now, let us look at what creates a fantastic start to the day. The way we start something sets a precedent for the rest of the day. Upon waking, we should get out of bed within five seconds. No snoozing, no excuses, no playing on your phone. Get up, drink a big glass of water, brush your teeth, wash your face, and then begin the following activities: silence (meditation or deep breathing to provide clarity); affirmations (self-talk); write down what you want to achieve (short-term, medium-term and long-term goals); visualisation (imagine what you want in your life); exercise (it reduces stress, boosts energy and ensures mental sharpness); reading (study things that are important to you); write (this can be notes, writing up a to-do-list, writing in your journal, writing a book, writing down what you are grateful for etc.) Take the first two hours of your day very seriously. You will notice that you become so much more productive. These first few hours of your day compound over time, so that you can create the kind of inner and outer strength you desire.

In addition, establish a quality nighttime routine. Not only is it really good for your health, but it makes us feel more in control before we sleep. Finishing the day with a nice routine prepares the mind for a restful sleep. It also builds consistency and trust within you. So what is a great nighttime routine? Start with a shower (preferably alternating with hot and cold water), and apply a quality shower gel to nourish your skin. Then apply a nutrient-dense lotion all over the body. Next, apply a nighttime face moisturiser. After that, brush your teeth thoughtfully. Subsequently, plan the tasks and your short-term goals for the following day as this enables you to start the next day with clarity and direction. The penultimate thing you may wish to do is read over anything imperative that you need to memorise or remember. Before you get into bed, you may want to take essential supplements such as vitamin D3, magnesium and fish oils, so that they provide your body with key nutrients whilst you sleep and recover. You may even want to sip apple cider vinegar as it is healthy and supports quality sleep. There you have it. A brilliant start and end to a productive day. It ends with you feeling physically and mentally stronger. This will create the kind of discipline and power needed to go for what you want. Improve the quality of your overall life, and watch the beautiful things open up to you in a plethora of ways. Something tells me you will be sleeping even better now.

We must use our time effectively. We should understand when our brain and body work best during the day, and dedicate that time to complete the most meaningful tasks. Whatever takes precedence needs to be given the right time and energy. For example, if you are a morning person, then set aside the pertinent time required in the morning to get these most difficult and important tasks done, and vice versa. Attack these tasks when you have the most energy and enthusiasm. This effective use of time makes you feel more competent, thereby developing your self-esteem, which affects your decisions as the rest of the day unfolds (resulting in healthier life choices).

Daily Exercise

Instil the habit of exercising every single day! Every single person, if physically capable, should be able to exercise between 10-20 minutes each day. Keeping the body active and moving is fantastic for our metabolism, and to constantly burn those extra calories. Every little bit accumulates. Have certain mini workouts that you can do every single day without even needing to go to the gym. Identify what exercises you love to do, and rely on these especially on days when you do not feel up for training. Even if you know you do not feel up for training, make sure you do something! It is all about momentum and consistency.

Whilst it is imperative to exercise every day, it is equally important to know when to train intensely, and when to take it easy when exercising. Save your most intense workouts for your days off work, or for your less hectic days at work. Whilst it is important to enjoy exercising, if we want to really see physical improvements then we must do the exercises that we least enjoy doing: they tend to be the exercises, and muscles, we most neglect and feel less competent when performing. Know when to pace yourself, and when to go hard in the gym. Listen to your body. It is not about proving how tough we are to others or ourselves. Be wise. Plan out your schedule. We mush decide when to train intensely, and when we should lower the intensity. Know your body well. Know how you feel after certain workouts. Know how quickly or slowly your body becomes sore and recovers after an intense workout. How can you exercise more intelligently? The more we over train, the worse we feel, and thus the more susceptible we become to wanting to eat even more and usually the wrong type of foods.

If we train between 60%-75% of our maximum capacity every day, then we do wonders for our metabolism, our congruency and our fat-loss endeavours. Our bodies soon require and need this activeness because of the positive releases experienced, and for the gradual benefits we will notice physically. If we train less than 60% of our best, then we risk not jumpstarting our metabolism for the day: the exercise then becomes more of a dynamic stretch, which is still good of course but not what we are aiming for if we are setting high standards. If we train over 75% every single day, then we will obviously over train, and our bodies will not be able to recover or function well consistently.

Eat Simple Meals Daily

Activities will remain consistent if they are easy to follow. This is even more important when it comes to our eating schedule. Most days should consist of similar meals and at similar times where possible. Know what foods you like; know what foods you would be happy to eat on most days, and choose meals that are relatively easy to prepare. The easier the process, the easier it is to understand and follow. It is similar to why Steve Jobs wore the same outfit every day. It simplifies the whole process. You do not have to think about what you must eat, and what you must prepare because you already know the procedure!

The simpler we make things for ourselves, the less tension (stress) we accumulate, which conspicuously affects our emotions, and thus how we eat. Too much choice makes it harder to choose, and thus we end up going down different paths (often paths that work against our fat-loss goals). When we have a rigid plan for our eating and training, then we cut out the garbage (no pun intended). If one domino falls, then it has a colossal knock-on effect on the others. This is how our health operates. We must come up with a winning formula (the routines we do every day that keeps us on track), and we must do these as often as possible. This is how we create long-term success. Over time, these routines become easier, and they do not feel burdensome. We are subsequently in a stronger position to take on newer routines, exercises and disciplines that compound our progress.

We are likely to go through phases in terms of what type of meals we prefer, and we are likely to make small adaptations to our meals over time. It might be helpful to write down three different possible options to have for your first meal of the day. Have another three meals to potentially choose from for lunch, and then have three meals to choose from for dinner. This makes it nine different meals that we can choose from every day. Feel free to change these nine options once every few months in order to provide some kind of variety. Moreover, the body becomes accustomed to eating certain foods consistently, so we benefit in many ways by alternating these every now and then. These nine meals can be chosen depending on the time of year, and what your goals are: purely for fat loss or muscle gain.

Cold Showers

"A morning contrast shower works as a gym, sauna and spa in your bathroom." - Stan Jacobs

Firstly, cold showers can condition our nervous systems to be more resilient when it comes to stress. Over time, our bodies adjust to the healthy oxidative stress that cold showers put on our nervous systems. Cold showers are probably the best way to learn how to focus and stay positive. Every single one of us initially reacts to extreme cold-water exposure the same way: we want to get out! However, the more experienced we become, the more we learn how to actually breathe better in these cold showers; we learn to actually think normally and not let things negatively affect us when in and out of the shower. We have conditioned ourselves to be stronger and more emotionally resilient. This directly transcends into positively affecting our discipline as it relates to pushing ourselves in the gym, and to make better food-related decisions.

Cold showers have been shown to increase our alertness and energy. Intriguingly, the drastic changes that occur to our breathing when having a cold shower is an attempt to keep the body warm due to the shock of the freezing cold water. It forces us to increase our oxygen intake, which has a very therapeutic effect on us. It does wonders for our energy levels, which is exactly what we need to think positively more often, and thus make better choices for our health: everyone makes smarter choices when they feel strong and energetic. Moreover, cold showers support blood circulation and immunity. The increase in our heart rate ensures that our blood circulates our body more rapidly, thereby helping to eliminate additional toxins. It can encourage blood to surround our organs. Additionally, the cold ensures strong blood circulation, helping arteries to competently pump blood, which can help with our immune system as well as with lowering our blood pressure.

In addition, cold showers can be very effective for reducing muscle soreness and speeding up muscle recovery. Cold-water exposure, especially over 20 minutes worth, can relieve muscle soreness for between one to four days after strenuous exercise. This is great for keeping us on track when it comes to training more often, but it also helps us to make better choices as it relates to our nutrition and consumption because we tend to eat more unhealthily when over trained and sore. It is a reaction to try and help us recover more quickly, which ends up becoming counterproductive. Unsurprisingly, cold showers also directly encourage fat loss. We activate our brown fat, 'good fat,' which functions to warm us up when exposed to intense cold. Cold showers therefore keep our brown fat active, enabling us to lose those extra pounds of fat the more we utilise cold-shock therapy.

As you can imagine, these physical adaptations when having cold baths or showers also help to reduce uric acid levels whilst improving Glutathione levels in our blood, which makes us less stressed generally. The more we reduce our stress levels, the more in control we feel. It becomes that much easier for us to eat more healthily. Moreover, cold showers have been shown to relieve depression as it stimulates the brain's major source of noradrenaline, which functions to alleviate depression. The positive shock delivered to the brain during a cold shower sends copious electrical impulses from peripheral nerve endings to the brain. In short, extreme cold exposure can improve our wellbeing.

Incantations and Anchoring

"NOW I AM THE VOICE. I WILL LEAD NOT FOLLOW. I WILL BELIEVE, NOT DOUBT. I WILL CREATE, NOT DESTROY. I AM A FORCE FOR GOOD. I AM A FORCE FOR GOD. I AM A LEADER. DEFY THE ODDS. SET A NEW STANDARD. STEP UP!" - Tony Robbins

Our healthy-eating plans will be tested every single day whether it is by friends, businesses, our peers or ourselves. We must be able to use affirmations (repeating an idea or belief to get a certain result) and incantations (using our physical movements and gestures along with saying these ideas or beliefs intensely to get a certain result) whenever we are feeling like we crave something unhealthy. We must embed powerful sayings within us that we turn to such as, "I am stronger than this," or "I know this trick, and I will stay on the right path," or "I am in charge of what I eat." Have a select few statements that you can memorise and use whenever you feel that you must change your state.

Incantations are extremely powerful in generating the level of focus, intensity and peak states that we require. We can condition ourselves (anchoring) to feel a certain way immediately because of what we associate mentally and emotionally to a physical action. If we repetitiously say something powerful intensely enough whilst we carry out the same physical action, then we can learn to trigger an automatic response (an anchor) at will. This tool is invaluable. It will keep you on track in moments of uncertainty and poor-quality states. It can trigger positivity and power within, so that we consistently make the right choices.

We can condition ourselves to access powerful, uplifting and supportive states. What can you do as your action? It depends on what you want to feel. Do you want to feel calmer? Do you want to feel stronger? Do you want to feel passionate? What do you do whenever you win at something, or whenever you want to get your focus back on track? Do you click your fingers? Do you smack your chest? Do you make a fist and shout "yes?" Do you smile and laugh? Do you pray? Your action can actually be far less obvious especially if it is inappropriate to do some of these actions in the workplace for instance! For example, you can just hold your right wrist with your left hand more tightly, or you can covertly just tug on your ear. If you have chosen a rather active move, then you can always perform this in your office or in the restroom etc. Decide on your action now.

Consider what you want to say to yourself when doing this manoeuvre. Keep it short, concise, use emotive words and include an "I am" that is positively phrased. For example, "I am ready to deliver at the highest level," or "I am ready to give myself to you Lord/Allah to do what I must with all my strength," or "I am a winner," or "I am deserving of any and all magnificent things that are about to happen." It is also worth considering your breathing in these states. How do you want to breathe? This goes back to what state you want to create. If you want to feel passionate and intense, then take fast and ferocious breaths. If you want to remain calm, then take deep inhales and even deeper exhales. Additionally, here are some other variable to consider: Where do you look, and how do you look? What are you thinking about when in these states? Do you think more or less? What kind of voice are you hearing in your head during these moments? Is it loud and powerful or clear and calm? What are your internal representations?

Lastly, we may even want to visualise either how we want to look or be. We can also remember past experiences where we did things brilliantly or when we were proud of our accomplishments. Once we have chosen a specific action (anchor), saying (affirmation) and visualisation, then we must practice it over and over again until the pattern is engrained within us. Whenever we perform it, however, we must do so with absolute belief and commitment. Really go for it. This creates the kind of energy and fortitude to really communicate things to yourself, and thus others, with the enthusiasm, passion and determination we need.

Breathe

"If you want to conquer the anxiety of life, live in the moment, live in the breath." – Amit Ray

Starting your day with conscious breathing enables you to take control of the day. We set the tone for the rest of the day. By starting the day controlling our inner workings, our breathing in this instance, then we teach the mind that we will be in control of ourselves no matter what unfolds during the day. Conscious breathing teaches us to be in the present moment. We can change our breathing patterns whenever we feel like we crave something unhealthy. It can change our state, allowing us to stay calm and emotionally detached from making unhelpful food choices.

It may sound rather simplistic, but breathing is a fundamental component that cannot be overlooked. We can change our states and thoughts by manipulating our breathing. Breathing in different tempos, exertions, rhythms, and so on, can drastically change our states. In terms of forming a more serene and tranquil state, we will want to breath in for at least four seconds, through the stomach and not the chest, and then hold our breath for at least six seconds, and then we will want to exhale for at least eight seconds. We can build our tolerance over time, so there is no need to push yourself and make yourself uncomfortable. This form of breathing improves clarity, and relaxes us, enabling us to put things into perspective: not taking things too seriously as we see them for what they really are, which is a small problem in comparison to much larger concerns.

Breathing and cold therapy expert, Wim Hof, teaches a similar deep breathing method that is even more intense and profound. When lying down, with your back against the bed, simply practice breathing in and taking in as much oxygen as you possibly can. Even when you think you have breathed in as much as you can, then you can still take in some more gulps of air through your mouth and nose until you have fully maximised the space within. We will feel like a balloon that has be blown up to the maximum at this stage. Once we have done this, then we can begin to exhale, but we should only exhale the usual amount (not as though we are trying to drain every bit of oxygen out of our bodies). We should do this ten times and then that is a breathing set completed. Complete as many sets as you wish.

Whilst we can inhale and exhale deeply to relax us, we can also inhale and exhale more quickly and profusely, thereby dramatically changing our state and energy levels due to the high amount of oxygen being pumped in and the carbon dioxide being pushed out. This rapid form of breathing changes the body's and mind's rhythm and circulation. Also, it can be a great way of eliminating toxins within the body. This form of breathing can dramatically alter our states, and make us feel light headed, so be cautious and refrain from breathing like this when working with machinery or when driving etc.

The fitter we are, the more slowly we tend to breathe when resting generally, and the more slowly we breathe, the more relaxed we feel. Fitter individuals therefore feel more relaxed when doing their usual day-to-day tasks. Think about what this does to our stress levels and daily energy. Unhealthier individuals tend to breathe more fiercely and loudly when in more relaxed states (like they are struggling almost), which is a clear indicator that their lungs are not operating as efficiently as they could. Fitness levels are linked to calmness. Consider the following questions: How do you usually breathe? How do you breathe when you are totally confident and feeling powerful? How do you breathe when apprehensive? How do you breathe when you are with a good friend? How do you breathe when you read? Learn to be more conscious of your breathing throughout the day, as a way of manipulating your states and stress levels (stress is closely tied to how we eat).

Partaking in yoga can also be very beneficial for changing how we breathe generally. When we are moving and stretching during yoga, ensure that we breathe deeply with every movement we make. If we match our breaths with our movements, then we create physical and mental synchronicity. We want our internal processes (breathing) to be congruent with our externals (movements). This keeps us aligned. It makes us more centred, more in control and, therefore, more ready to effectively deal with the day's challenges and inevitable stresses. Meditation can also be wonderful. It is a great opportunity to practice positive thinking or to clear our minds. This sets a wonderful tone for the rest of the day.

Just Do It

One of the best psychological strategies we can utilise on a daily basis is to simply do what we must without thinking about it. The moment we hesitate, the more space we create between the activity and us. If we know we must do something, then do not allow ourselves to overthink and rationalise. We run the risk of putting ourselves off. I am a massive fan of intermittent fasting, abstaining from consuming any form of calories for 16 hours and above several times per week. The later we wait into our fast before we do our exercise, the better it is for our fat loss. You can imagine how easy it must be to convince yourself to just start eating after you have been working during the day, but really what I want to do is go straight to the gym after I have completed most of my work for the day. At that point, the mind is more vulnerable and susceptible to empathetic talk, and because I know that it is easy to talk myself out of going to the gym at this point, I now do not make it an option. If you give yourself an option to pull out, then we will pull out more often than not. This is why we must simply get changed into our gym wear and just show up! It does not matter if you do not train intensely and feel incredible. You will notice, that you become less hungry when the body starts moving and when the mind gets focuses on training and not food when in the gym. Excuses are always there. We must be strong enough to suffocate its self-sabotaging sayings.

Blind Spots

We usually do not have to eat the last snack or meal of the day. Everyone's mind works differently. Some people are stronger mentally in certain situations, and not as strong in other psychological areas. I have noticed that my own personal 'blind spot' occurs right at the end of most days. For instance, I usually utilise intermittent fasting, and when it comes to the evening, I usually eat quite a bit as you can imagine. Once I have enjoyed my dinner, I should ideally refrain from eating anything, and go to bed. Without fail, I will have my self-sabotaging voice throw its two pence in: "Just eat another snack. You've been awesome all day. You will fast again tomorrow, so you are going to struggle unless you eat a bit more." Through experience, I have learned that this is not the case. My challenge is to ensure that the last thing I eat is my dinner, and that is it. When I eliminate that last snack, even if it is not necessarily unhealthy, I notice a drastic change in my fat loss. Small things accumulate. Those last couple hundred calories taken away on most days really make a huge difference. Consider your 'blind spot.' What is the biggest challenge you encounter almost every day that could be ruining your body-shape goals? Do you convince yourself that a certain treat is quite healthy when in reality it is not? Do you always find a way to justify eating a certain thing or at a certain time? Do you excuse yourself from exercising in the morning because you have convinced yourself that an extra hour of sleep is more 'beneficial?' Write out these limiting beliefs, and break them down one by one. Dispel its power, and make the small shifts necessary to really get the body you deserve.

Transfer Successes

Think about something that you do very well. It does not have to be related to health or physical aspirations. Maybe you are doing brilliantly in your career. Maybe you have excellent relationships with friends. Maybe you have taken a hobby to the highest level. Maybe you are great at public speaking. Maybe you are superb at social networking. What makes you so successful in this area? I am sure that one of your strengths in this area is your ability to perceive it as a long-term task or goal. It is something you see yourself doing for many years if not decades. Think about what psychological tools you utilise, so that you remain on track every single day. We want to transfer these powerful thoughts and emotional patterns into the world of healthy eating and exercise.

What rules, tasks or obstacles do you encounter on a daily basis that could possibly prevent you from doing really well in this area? Compare the obstacles you face, with your current strength, and identify the similarities you encounter with healthy eating and exercise. What similarities are there? What differences are there? What phrases and words in your vocabulary can you transfer from your strength to the world of nutrition and exercise? We want to feel strong feelings of success with our strength, and feel the same way when we encounter matters relating to health and fitness. What do you think to yourself when partaking in your strong area? Think like this when deciding what to eat or if you should train. What do you feel when in your powerful state, and how can you transfer these to deciding what you eat or when you are training? How do you breathe before and during moments when you experience flow (your strength)? See if you can transfer this to your healthy experiences. How do you move before and during your strong experience? Can you display these same/similar movements to matters relating to health such as when you are going out to eat or when you are on your way to the gym? What is your focus when experiencing your strength? Can you display this same level of focus when you are eating healthily or when you are training hard at the gym? What are you certain of when experiencing your strengths? Could you display this same level of certainty and confidence when partaking in healthy habits? Take your energy, confidence and inner power from your strength, and directly transfer the same body language, internal representations and activeness into the world of healthy eating and exercise.

For example, even though I am generally a very calm, serene person, I am also very intense and passionate especially when partaking in some of the things that I do best. When at the gym, I am very expressive, I bounce around quite a bit and I have a very determined look. I will smile at others, be light on my feet, make a lot of eye contact, inhale and exhale quite deeply and powerfully, and I will invariably say many positive things to myself: "Let's do this." "Give everything that you have." "Enjoy every moment." "I am in my element." These are some of the sub-modalities and variables involved when I train. I have now taken many of these physical and mental traits, and I take them into an area that I have been working on recently such as when studying or writing about a new topic. It allows me to access my strongest states. Write down the things you think and physically do when in your peak state. Write down what aspects you can utilise when in the gym, preparing your meals and so on.

Be Specific

If we are to plan and execute better healthy routines, so that we come closer to transforming our bodies and health, then we must focus on one strategy at a time for many reasons: to avoid feeling overwhelmed; to focus on one thing at a time; to do this one step the best possible way. We want to focus on behavioural changes. Look to replace one unhealthy treat, or aspect of a meal, with a healthier replacement. Once this habit is instilled, then we can make the next change. Here are some specific examples of changes that can be made that are very clear and specific, and therefore we can always follow through with them. Example 1) Avoid the nighttime snack by having double portions of vegetables. Example 2) No sauces are to be added to meals. Example 3) Instead of eating huge meals, start each meal by drinking a big glass of water or with an apple. Example 4) Instead of having an unhealthy bar or treat, replace it with a health shake of some kind: with protein powder or a green shake. Take a moment to consider to small adjustments you can make, and create a weekly plan of the changes you will implement. Start with the easiest changes first, that you know you can succeed with in order to build momentum and self-belief. The moment you fail to implement what you thought was an already embedded habit, then refrain from continuing with your latest or next healthy habit, and go back a step. If you stick to the plan you have created, then success is inevitable. Veering off the plan will result in mental chaos, and a fight to juggle many balls that will seem insurmountable. Unfortunately, this only results in regression.

Conclusion

"We are what we repeatedly do. Excellence, therefore, is not an act but a habit." - Aristotle

All of the different aspects this book work synergistically to create the inner energy and strength needed to make better choices, not just for our bodies and health, but also in life generally. One of the elements that appeared frequently in several of these chapters was energy. We need energy to overpower our negativity; we need energy to keep active and focused on what we want to achieve; we need energy to resist the many temptations that are oftentimes just seconds away from harming us. We need energy to go to the gym; we need energy to complete projects; we need energy to communicate in our relationships. Do whatever you can to improve your energy levels, and you will see the benefits in all areas of your life. Avoid complacency because if we fall into this trap, then we will fail to grow, and, naturally, we will feel lazier, inactive and thus sad. Depression will then seep in, and then emotional eating will again take control. Tony Robbins shares that, "The strongest people are not those who show strength in front of us, but those who win battles we know nothing about." If we are to consistently succeed in terms of our daily habits, then we must feel strong internally. Feeling powerful is more about feeling strong enough to tackle any obstacles that come our way, and so power is more about how much energy we have on a daily basis. No one feels powerful mentally, emotionally or physically if they are frequently exhausted. Therefore, if we want to feel more powerful, then we have to partake in daily activities that enable us to grow and move closer to achieving our goals. Some of these activities include meditation/yoga, incantations, writing out our goals, doing things that take us closer to achieving our goals, exercising, sex and pushing our boundaries. The more flow we experience on a daily basis, the more powerful we feel. Flow is power.

Act with urgency in life. Life is short, and we all know how quickly time flies by. Achieve more now. Take action now. Love more now. We are on this earth, in our own unique form, for a blink of an eye. We are in charge of what we think, feel and create around us. The more loving and appreciative we are of ourselves, the more we partake in activities with clarity, self-respect and without judgement. Our daily lives determine how satisfied, energetic and passionate we are. So now that we have the knowledge, we must now take the information in these chapters, and engrain them within your subconscious. The only way to do this is to make them habitual. Lastly, I suggest that you read this book at least once a year to embed the notions explored, and as your life experiences change, you will perceive these ideas differently, and thus continue to make new insights from this book. Improving the quality of our lives is partly down to transferring more of our short-term thinking actions into long-term thinking actions. True happiness is about the emotions we experience daily, and whether we feel that our activities are taking us closer to where we want to be. Being focused on short-term gratification will result in long-term pain. Short-term thinkers are most likely to become impatient, addicts and people who struggle financially (rarely do get rich quick schemes ever work). Be a long-term thinker, but take action toward these long-term goals now and daily! Discipline is the most important skill needed in life. It is not talent or ability. Do things every day to keep yourself on track.

We have the ability to improve all our strengths and all our weaknesses. We must develop a growth mindset. Ask the right questions, and search for the right answers. We must treat our lives like a computer game: we want to be in control of what we do and when we do them as much as possible. We also want to remain detached, so that we make better decisions more often rather than being swayed by the emotions of our egos. A balance between giving the ego expression, yet remaining detached from our experiences is essential. There is no need to force anything in life. All we need to do is develop our character, mentality and spirit, and watch how the seemingly impossible become possible.

What is your endgame? How do you know if you have lived a fulfilling life? Isn't that the real definition of success? Success, and being a winner in life, is about living a long, healthy and exciting life. These three constituents encapsulate the meaning of success and happiness. Self-esteem refers to our ability to think what we choose to think without letting anybody dictate our inner processes. Amusingly, there is no moment where we will feel completely successful; happiness is an ongoing process. There is no line that we pass that ascertains whether we are happy. We may think that a great body is what we really want in life, but what we really want is to feel loved and happy within ourselves. The process of life, and the entire journey, provides happiness. Happiness never arrives. This is one of life's biggest illusions. Life is a game; we must create our own stipulations for this game. In many ways, to remain focused on what is important in life, such as our health and physiques, it is always beneficial to start from the end, and work our way down: imagine yourself as an old man or woman. What kind of example do you want to have set for those who are close to you? What would you have wanted to achieve as an elderly person? How do you want your friends, children and grandchildren to remember you? How can you begin to condition this now? What will you need to accomplish? How can this be done?

Living healthily is not about avoiding errors (as these are inevitable to an extent); it is about how quickly we can recover from our errors, and it is about learning from them. We can liken success in terms of our health and body to the art of boxing. Problems and obstacles are always going to hit us. We simply cannot avoid some small and huge problems. No one is skilled enough to evade the punches that life will throw at us. However, people react in one of two ways when a problem is launched at them. Firstly, let us look at how not to take a punchy problem: the problems that knock us out are the ones that we do not see coming. We may be so blinded by our egos that we get caught off guard. We have been ignoring life's jabs (warnings) so often that we somehow allowed ourselves to get hit by the power shot. Life's punches also knock people flat when people brawl in life as opposed to developing technique and avoiding unnecessary punishment (problems). What do we mean by brawling? We mean just banking on being tough, and thinking that toughness is enough. Being a fighter will help you survive, but we are after the victory! Giving what we have and risking getting hit a lot is a recipe for disaster!

We can only take so many blows until the strength of our 'chin' diminishes. It then becomes easier for life to overwhelm us. There is only so much we can handle in life. We must play it smart. We must pick our moments. We must be patient. We must attack when the time is right. Since we cannot duck, slip and roll from all punches thrown at us, we need to learn how to roll with the punches. It means we must anticipate what problems might occur and when; we must be able to move our faces with the opponent's punch, so that we take some of the force off the punch. If we take a punch full on, then we will get hurt badly, which is what most reactive people feel: the short-term thinker. If we try to walk through the punch, then life's problems will catch up on us. If we think a punch coming, and yet we move toward it (focusing on the negatives in our lives), then the inevitable will happen. However, being proactive, and developing our defense, will keep us protected, so that we can pick our shots when opportunities present themselves.

Our levels of success in terms of our body shape, overall health and happiness are dependent upon our emotional intelligence. Being able to influence yourself will greatly affect your feelings of success most dramatically. Being able to influence yourself means knowing how to get yourself to take the action required consistently. It means knowing how to find the right kind of leverage to play with our own emotions in a way to get the best out of us, and this can happen in different ways. Being able to influence others is mandatory if we are to keep everyone at the right length, whether close or far, so that we can focus on our biggest life goals such as our health and energy. We want to experience mostly positive feelings every day, and we want to have copious energy every day.

Positivity + Energy = Your Ideal Health and Body

We must believe that we deserve great health and a stunning body. We must believe that we are enough just as we are now. We must believe that life will unfold the way we wish, as long as we keep pressing forward diligently. Lastly, we must be ourselves, and live abundantly: give more, love more and focus on what we want more. I wish you all the physical and mental success in the world, and I hope this book brings you great pleasure and self-esteem.

Bibliography

Hall, Michael. *Meta States: Mastering the Higher Levels of Your Mind.* Neuro-Semantic Publications. 2009.

Bandler, Richard. *Get the Life You Want: The Secrets to Quick & Lasting Life Change.* Harper Element. 2008.

Byrne, Rhonda. *The Secret.* Beyond Words Publishing. 2006.

Dweck, Carol. *Mindset: The New Psychology of Success.* Ballantine Books. 2006.

Elrod, Hal. *The Miracle Morning: The 6 Habits That Will Transform Your Life Before 8AM.* John Murray Learning. 2012.

Peters, Steve. *The Chimp Paradox: The Mind Management Programme to Help You Achieve Success, Confidence and Happiness*. Penguin Books. 2012.

Robbins, Anthony. *Unlimited Power: The New Science of Personal Achievement*. Pocket Books. 2001.

Tzu, Lao. *Tao Te Ching*. Hackett Classics. 1993.

Printed in Great Britain
by Amazon